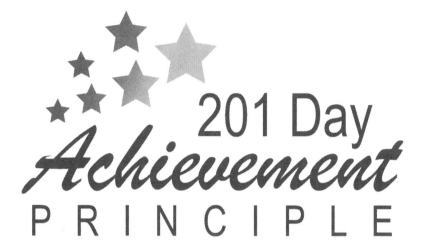

201 Day
Achievement
P R I N C I P L E

Join the movement and accomplish your goals by establishing fulfilling practices, applying realistic commitments, and ensuring consistent tracking.

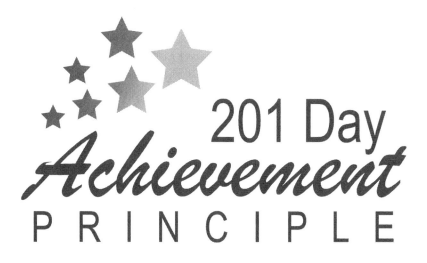

201 Day
Achievement
P R I N C I P L E

Your journey to freedom through conscious choice

Kim White and Teresa Easler

This book is printed on acid-free paper.
Publication date March 2020.
Version 1.0
ISBN-9781661859572

Book Design by Theresa McNeilly of DoTheWorkBooks.com
Logo Design by Bruce Canales of BrandanaMarketing.com

To order your copy of the 201 Day Achievement Principle, visit us at
www.201dayachievementprinciple.com

We have created an online community where you can engage with others, make connections, become encouraged to continue, find an accountability partner, share experiences, and elicit and provide feedback.

Community is critical for significant transformation when following through with any new goal, practice, or challenge. We'll be there as well to help support and encourage you.

Join us now on Facebook
Facebook/201 Day Achievement Principle

Connect with us on Instagram
Instagram@201DayAchievementPrinciple

and feel free to send us direct messages through
201dayachievementprinciple@connecttothecore.com

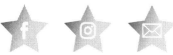

Download this FREE breakthrough worksheet to begin your journey with the 201 Day Achievement Principle

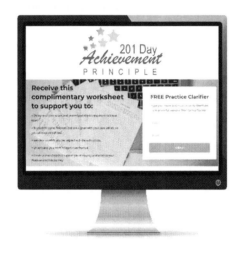

☆ Define your core values and understand why it's important to know them

☆ Brainstorm some Practices that are aligned with your core values so you can become fulfilled

☆ Get clear on WHY you feel aligned with those Practices and understand your WHY for each new Practice

☆ Create a vision board to support you in staying connected to your Practices and this journey

Sign up for this free worksheet at 201dayachievementprinciple.com

**Stay on TRACK with the
201 Day Achievement Principle
with these Tracking Tools**

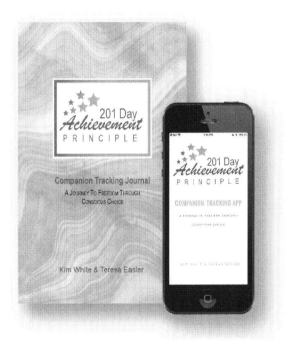

☆ Use the 201 Day Achievement Principle Tracking Journal to keep track, take notes and record celebrations

☆ Use the 201 Day Achievement Principle App to send you reminders everyday

**To order your Tracking Journal or
to download the App go to
201dayachievementprinciple.com**

Contents

OUR STORY

Kim

When I was a child, during the 60's and 70's, running was pure joy for me. Any chance I got to run, I would; especially zooming around corners. Fast forward to 1992, during my Olympic training, I was running fourteen times a week. Then, due to injury I retired from professional running. I had become overwhelmed by my passion and lost my joy to run.

It wasn't until the early 2000's that I began to look to running again—this time as a solution for my health. I was getting short of breath, I'd put on a lot of weight, and found it hard to bend over and tie my laces.

So I created a goal to run a few times a week. Over the next few years I tracked my running which turned out to be 80-150 days a year. In 2011, I decided I wanted to run more than that, so I set a goal to run 200 days in a year. There was one rule: I wasn't going to force myself. In 2016, I ran 201 days—55%—of the year. That number felt good with me. I totally enjoyed the process. I celebrated and posted it on Facebook. I knew I was on to something. Tracking the practice with 201 out of 365 as a goal was what I needed—success without stress or pressure.

As a result of reading my post, some of my old running buddies decided to 'establish a practice and track their participation'. The system worked fantastically, and the group support and accountability was a bonus.

With no pressure to run every day, and the system in place to maintain my 201/365 goal, I started to lose weight, feel stronger, think more clearly, and really enjoy it, just like I did when I was a kid.

My wish for you is that you find joy in the practices you want to do for 201 days out of 365—physically, mentally, emotionally, spiritually... the sky's the limit. Enjoy your journey.

Kim White

Teresa

A few years ago I was feeling 'off track' with some of my regular practices—yoga and meditation, in particular. I was hard on myself when I didn't do these things every day. I saw success as all or nothing. This created inner-tension; the 'missing days' drove me into a negative mindset.

Meet my dear friend Kim White. I saw he'd posted on Facebook that he'd just completed his 201st run of the year. I had two immediate thoughts. Firstly, Wow! Running 201 times in a year is pretty great and, secondly, he had kept track of it. I thought about how, over time, I'd let something I loved and wanted to do—yoga—slip. I decided to apply Kim's magic number to it. His formula worked. Success followed, and I soon added other practices I wanted to do more of—such as meditation, and abstinence from sugar and flour.

I have said—partially in jest—that the preparation for my choices took place over thirty years. I want to make sure people don't need thirty years. This book will ensure that no one will.

My wish is that you experience the freedom and breakthroughs that come with prioritizing the things that are most important to you. I am excited for each person to experience their 'aha!' when learning that freedom of choice and success go hand in hand.

Teresa B. Easler

★ ★ ★ ★ ★

Inspiration is a remarkable growth-inducing kind of thing. When we saw the power in choosing a practice and tracking that practice, and when we tested it with others and saw the value in support and sharing, we knew we had to tell the world—after all, we are people persons. We put our heads together and:

☆ assembled a phenomenal team

☆ brainstormed

☆ invented a tracking journal

☆ began a pilot group

☆ set up a support system

☆ listened to the participants

☆ gathered data

☆ improved the tracking journal

☆ created an app

We went on to discover that while achieving 55% offered a great psychological boost, there were still benefits noted when people rolled in under 55%. Whether the practices chosen were related to business or personal, selecting a practice (or two or three or five) based on want, choosing when to do it, and tracking it consistently, caused the earth to move under the feet of our pilot participants.

We put our findings in a book—this book—to support the tracking journal. Now people from all walks of life can fully understand and celebrate the freedom that comes from the choice of 'doing' or 'not doing' a daily practice. We want people to experience the positive outcomes that are consequences of tracking their practices. We even created a global community of likeminded practice-ers to become inspirers and/or to receive support.

Kim & *Teresa*

YOUR STORY

Yes, your story, and why not? You are as much a part of this book as its creators. You are its co-creator by way of contributing as a reader and through being a participant in the process.

No matter your situation, your age, occupation, or state of health, you belong here. Everybody belongs.

Activation in the project began when you purchased your book. It continues with your input in this book and in the journal. You are, after all, the author of your own life.

Some people are good just to 'think' their thoughts and answers, others find it helpful to record them. Either way, on a joint venture like this one, we all need a bit more space to stretch out than is provided in the margins. You'll find that space throughout this book.

This book will become the foundation for new thoughts and considerations. If you have said or thought any of the following, get ready to achieve success through a different approach.

☆ I've tried other 'things' before and they haven't stuck.

☆ I want to believe in myself.

☆ I have specific goals I've wanted to reach for some time.

☆ I need a simple system that works.

☆ I want to stop beating myself up about lack of consistency.

☆ There's a creative genius in me waiting to jump out past the procrastinator.

☆ I am a 'don't have enough time' kind of person.

Get ready to discover how 201 Day Achievement Principle promotes success and removes the pressure of 'the streak'—the all or nothing.

Coming Face-to-Face With Yourself Before You Dive In.

Before I get into focusing on what practices I will choose, before I learn about what a practice is, here's what I know about me.

I picked this book up because

The biggest challenge in my life is

If I were to put a star on the fridge for something I do, I am, or have achieved, what would it be for?

Words I use to describe myself

Words others use to describe me

Three wishes for myself

Anything else about me I want to express

INTRODUCTION

Train tracks lead to chosen destinations—exotic and exciting places waiting for travellers to arrive. There are express routes, which whiz by on non-stop schedules, blurring the scenery—sometimes those trips leave folks dizzied and out of breath. They seem to punctuate, even accentuate, the chaotic and fast-pace of a busy life. Thank goodness for scenic routes which stop at interesting places, offer the time and views that allow each traveler to experience a wider swath of the world, and to gather an understanding of the space between start and finish.

From start to finish, be it through the rails and the recording of platforms at stations, tracking a package from sender to recipient, or even following a first draft to final manuscript through an editor's track changes in electronic copy, all tracks and tracking lead to an outcome—a sensational destination, a long awaited package, or a book.

Keeping track of participation in an activity is vital to the generation of motivation. The regular recording of yes or no, in relation to having done something that moves people closer to a goal, is imperitive for success.

The 201 Day Achievement Principle came out of the recognition that the accomplishment of a goal—a desired or chosen outcome—was more achievable when thought and awareness were applied to the choice and the execution. The attainment of that goal, or mastery of that skill, was made a more enjoyable ride by marrying three components: selecting a practice that is a want, freely choosing when to work on it, and consistently tracking when it is worked on.

The 201 Day Achievement Principle discourages obsession and being fanatical. Skills are learned, goals are moved toward and accomplished through consistency laced with freedom.

In a way, moving toward 201/365 is like riding on a train: those steel rails keeping the engine, cars, and caboose on schedule and on the right route. With 201 Day Achievement Principle, there's time to enjoy the view from the window of the comfortable compartment. In selecting a trip to 'Any Station Except Should', there's a feel of holding a Golden Ticket to 'Accomplished What I Wanted'.

The 201 Day Achievement Principle is essentially your Golden Ticket.

In order to support you, and offer you the maximum opportunity for success, the presentation order and chapter content has been diligently evaluated by a diverse team of practice-ers. Composed to be as brief and impactful as possible, suited to a wide range of readers and learners, the components: CHOOSING, TRACKING, PRACTICING have been organized to inform and incite.

With the Golden Ticket in hand, YOU hold all the power.

We mostly approach things alone and throw ourselves into them rather than create a structure. 201 Day Achievement Principle is different than any other program you've encountered. No one is demanding one hundred percent participation. The fact that no one is demanding stringent perfection means you are likely to arrive at your year end as a changed person. You are choosing your goals and the amount of time you will practice in each session, as well as when you will practice. You hold all the power.

PART I

Choosing

"Be the leader of your life. You are the one in charge of your circumstances."

Teresa Easler

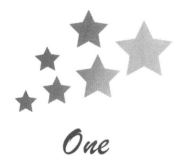

One

CLARIFICATION OF CHOICE-
PRACTICE VERSUS HABIT

People often confuse practice with habit. They are as different as being awake and asleep, conscious and unconscious.

Practices

Practices are things people 'consider' and 'think about' before doing them.

For the purpose of this book, practices are the things folks want to do more of, things around which people want to build skills, and excel at them.

Even when practices are ritualized—when someone has made space and time for them on a regular basis—they rarely become habit.

If a person wants to learn to speak German, the learning of German is a practice in which the 'student' progresses until fluent in the language.

If a person wants to write a book, the lead-up to learning how to write and putting words on paper is a practice. When the book is finished, the practice of writing other books can continue.

A practice is a decided-upon-in-a-time-frame act of doing and participating in a desired activity. It may be done often. It may be done on a schedule. But as long as there is a conscious decision to do it, it is a practice.

When you practice something, you make a conscious choice that begins with choosing the 'something' and choosing when to do that 'something'.

Habits

Habits are established routines that are seemingly involuntary.

Teeth brushing is a habit. Not one person says, 'I think I'll choose to brush my teeth today.' It is an automatic go-to-and-do in the morning and before bed. For some it's even rote between meals. Teeth brushing examples the epitome of habit.

Teeth brushing never ends.

Face washing never stops.

Hair brushing takes place every day.

Some will never *not* make the bed immediately after rising.

A habit is as close to the involuntary act of breathing as can be. It is accepted that when people do something out of habit they are unconsciously carrying out the action—seemingly as close to involuntarily as can be.

How many of us appear at breakfast, not even having registered that we have made the bed, combed our hair, or brushed our teeth? This is the key identifier of habit: we don't think about doing it and we often don't remember if we did.

Grey Zones Sorted

One way—albeit an extreme example—that brushing teeth could be a practice is if a person was raised by wolves and had never been exposed to dental hygiene, then entered society, and had to learn to get used to brushing his teeth twice a day. There would be reminders, there would be demonstrations. It would take a long time for the person to 'possibly' reach for the toothbrush without thinking.

You have always brushed your hair in the morning—side part, get rid of the tangles—just like your mother showed you when you were a toddler. Then, one day, you may have made a conscious choice to style your hair a certain way, a different way than usual. Perhaps you chose to go to a class or watched an online video to learn to braid your hair. That is a practice. You still step up to the mirror and brush your hair each morning (habit) but then you make the added choice to style it in a particular way. It would only be after years—decades perhaps—of braiding it daily that it might become habit-like.

The differentiation between habit and practice is the level of awareness of thought put into the action that follows.

"A year from now, what practice will I wish I had started today?"

Kim White

Two

A WORLD WITHOUT SHOULDING

Welcome to 201 Day Achievement Principle. The first rule of 201 Day Achievement Principle is: Do not 'should' your practice. The second rule of 201 Day Achievement Principle is: DO NOT 'SHOULD' YOUR PRACTICE! The final rule is: Always CHOOSE your practice.

Practices are never shoulds. If there is a hint of 'I should do this' in selecting your practice, it is the wrong practice; you are likely not looking at that practice in a healthy way that will benefit you and bring you success.

The thing is, we are caught up in a world of should haves; seduced by promise, then blasted by demands: try this, do that, come on, keep up. We regularly confuse what we ought to do with what we want to do.

Is it any wonder? Expectations flood our lives: create a website in a day, write a novel in a weekend, get in shape in thirty days— never has it been easier to take free online courses on any topic, and never has the pressure been higher over why people **should**. And when they don't—create that website or write that bestseller, or achieve some prescribed level of fitness—they experience guilt. "Why didn't I do it? What is wrong with me? Everyone else seems to be checking off items on a goal chart or bucket list. I **should** have worked on it yesterday."

Add to that the world of advertised self-objectivity: we are all bombarded with sponsored ads in social media that promise renewal, peace of mind, and financial windfalls. People click to find out their IQ, personality type, and what they will look like in twenty years, with an underlying belief those quizzes will create more self-knowledge. But, in reality, those bait and clicks mostly serve to capture electronic addresses.

A dozen invitations (to a webinar) later, and people are left wondering when they will find the backstage pass that will admit them to the 'real experience' that will show the way to reach those goals and desires long held close to the heart.

There's a lot of time spent (read: wasted) in dabbling in hopefulness and wishes. Now, that's different than dreaming—there's nothing wrong with dreaming. When wishes are dreamed in healthy doses it's the precursor to developing and doing.

Getting Out Of Your Own Way

We're all great at making lists: grocery, gift, chore, guest, and bucket. Who hasn't known the satisfaction of crossing off an item? But in reality, most of us do a lot of bringing forward, adding on, organizing, and revising columns of clutter. Folks swim in scraps of paper headed with 'to do', but when do any of us rise above and simply do—as in do what we want?

**Where is the list of the things you want to do?
And which of those things are you
actively and enjoyably practicing?**

It's easier to make a grocery list than a 'what I want to accomplish in life' list. Picking up eggs and apples is easily achieved. Successful are those who remember to grocery shop and then cross items off their list. The success rate is less when that item is to learn a language, walk a mile at lunchtime or, heaven forbid, consider the steps needed for a career change. Give me the eggs and the apples pick-up over that every time.

The thrill of crossing things off lists is universal. Check-marking all the items is the equivalent of receiving a star at the top of the paper—a throwback to primary school achievement.

But most of our lists—especially the bucket kind—end up explained away by: 'It's not-doable this month', 'It's complicated', 'Are you kidding me? I'm too stressed'. That mindset is always controlled by an inner CEO that insists on ALL or NOTHING. A do it, or fail. With that attitude, it's no wonder many give up, and even more put their wants on permanent hold.

Please don't put your 'wants' on hold any longer. Things are about to change. There is a much better place than ALL or NOTHING.

That place is found in the land of Choice which shares its border with Tracking and Practicing. And because of the terrain—in order to prepare you to choose wisely—we must go through Choice first.

The things you want to do are never shoulds. The practices you consider choosing will indicate your desire to grow, learn, have fun, engage... the key word here is desire. Your choice might be based on something you already do but are not doing as much of it as you want to, or it could be dipping your toe in the water of something you have never tried before. A world of success, reasonably and intelligently and consistently measured success, awaits you.

You Are More Than Worth It - You Are Worthy

We get out of life what we put into it. You already know that. It is the same with 201 Day Achievement Principle. That's why we want you to consider your choices carefully because this is not an 'I quit' program (because of its friendly 55% nature—more on the numbers in the tracking section). It is an 'I want to do it, I am doing it, I did it' program.

Must Be Clear On The Practice Chosen And Set The Session Times

You must want your 'want'. This cannot be emphasized enough. And your 'want' must be clearly defined. To want to knit or paint is a great 'want'. But why do you want to do either of these things? And, what will you knit or paint, where will you learn, what materials will you use, who will you knit or paint for? It is also essential to create a realistic time frame that will count as an official session—this also requires a lot of thought. It will differ for everyone. For example, drawing and sketching at home will not require transport to and from a classroom or studio. Forty-five minutes of beading might be harder on the eyes than thirty. An hour on the treadmill might be enough for one person but too much for another.

To come up with 'lose weight', and write 'diet' at the top of a page of any notebook, calendar, or tracking journal is beyond broad. To write 'Yoga' is extremely general. It's essential to be specific. The best outcomes are realized by being specific not only in the name you give to your practice, but in the 'why you want it' and 'how you will get it'. Ensuring your success is why this companion book—to the tracking journal—exists. We do not take your wants lightly, and neither should you. That's why we are stressing the importance of choice. You're going to be investing time in practices that will alter your life.

Your choice of wants or practices—and the way you express and define them—will substantially affect your outcome. The more succinct, the more personalized, the more 'thought out', the more likely you'll be in carrying out your practice 201 days (or more) out of 365.

Clarity = Success

Practices cover the gamut of desires. One person's desire is another person's 'no way'. As long as it's not a 'should' for you, then it is totally available as a choice. Further on, we've made a list of 201 practices that might rev your imagination.

Once you know your choice is not a should, then it's essential to clarify it. Does soap making mean taking a class at a community college or getting a book and winging it at home? Does it involve cleaning out a workspace or do you already have a spot?

This kind of clarity will become important when you assign times to practicing your practices.

Health goals and desires are not off limits. Again, as long as they're genuine wants they are totally practice-able. Clarity is key here too. For example, you may choose to aim for 201 days out of 365 of no dairy. If you review your whys (perhaps you've had some allergic symptoms), then you might want to abstain from dairy as your practice. (It makes sense. You'll be healthier. You may stop itching.) But if you think further—in the realm of clarity—butter is dairy, yogurt is dairy, milk is obviously dairy, and so is cheese that's on pizza and other foods you might love. There are several ways you can go here. Choose one 'general' practice—abstain from all dairy. Or separate them. You might then end up with abstaining from cheese, milk, butter, yogurt—four separate practices. This gives you the opportunity to be successful in one, two, three, or four things, rather than unsuccessful in a broader one.

By encouraging you to narrow your choice(s)—call it niching your practices—we're advocating for you to think, clarify, and set yourself up for success.

On this note, The Harvard Business Review shared some points as a result of extensive studies on motivation and goal setting. It's no surprise that their first point is to be precise. Summarized and paraphrased:

Specificity

Be sure of what it is you want. When you are sure of that 'want' then write it out, publicize it even, so that you are clear it is your 'want' or 'goal'. The absence of goals (or choosing to neglect an identified goal) is like walking backwards. You're moving your legs, but not moving forward.

Check Your Progress

Reward yourself, beyond the dopamine delivery you'll receive. Set milestones that act as measure of your performance. Short term targets deserve rewards. Rewards motivate.

Talk With Someone You Trust

There's nothing like a trusted mentor's take on things to straighten up your thinking and alter your actions. Self-reliance is great, but people don't always have the necessary self-control they think they will have. Turning to someone you have confidence in will give you the opportunity to 'hear' the other side of things—the view from 'their' perspective. A view not visible to you. It's a brilliant moment when a trusted friend can shed light and reveal one of your blind spots.

Have Fun, But Be Logical – Be Analytical
One of the best things you can do when there is a little confusion over what's important to you, even the little things (because little things become big things/big things are a bunch of little things), is to remain logical. To pause and evaluate. There is a lot to be said for taking time to yourself and focusing on your decisions. And lighten up. Logical doesn't prohibit laughter.

We think Harvard's observations are spot-on. Take the dairy example. Imagine if the decision was to abstain from all dairy without considering it could be split into a variety of groups. Part way through your year you might have discovered that you are abstaining from all except butter. You might have some regret. Not that you couldn't change it and establish new categories. This is only one example. The need to get serious and focus on the way you will define your want, and the journey there, is because your time is valuable. To arrive at your desired destination, to meet or exceed your target, is directly related to the way you set it all up. Set yourself up for success by taking the time to think about all the permutations of your 'want'.

The psychology of those stars you received on the stuff that went on the fridge is as significant today as it was in childhood. You have aged—but the psychology of reward remains the same. People may appear super-sophisticated in a corporate world, but all folks crave positive attention and feed off positive reinforcement.

It is through identifying a want (or two or five) and clearly ensuring it is what you want, then tracking your journey to it, that you will inspire yourself (and others).

The Bottom Line

Yes, it can take time to clarify and arrive at a practice. Consider the extra time in asking the whys and hows, and even the niching of your practices, as a level of self-respect of your time, and being in the interest of your outcome. Clarity in choice is vital.

TAKEAWAYS

★ You deserve to desire.

★ Choose only wants, never shoulds.

★ There is a much better place than ALL or NOTHING.

★ Clarity is key.

FAQ

How will I know that this is different than other programs? What are the other components that will make this work?
We're glad you want to know it all, but it's impossible to put it all up front for you at the same time. We hear your excitement—you probably can't wait to get going. That's a great sign. Don't worry, we'll get to the equally important part of tracking. It won't take long to fit the pieces together. You'll soon see what we mean by there's another place other than ALL or NOTHING. For now, ensure you read all about choice, focus on what it is you really want to do—one thing or more than one thing. And when you have that focus, make sure it's not a thing you've been told you should do.

LISTENING IN ON THE THOUGHTS OF OTHERS
INTERJECTION/EXCERPT:
A PARTICIPANT SHARES

"I thought about the word desire. I'd never associate that with 'should'. It reminded me of a phrase: top billing. I pictured a marquee outside an old fashioned movie house—my name next to a few star shapes. I thought to myself that it was time to put myself first in something I really want to do. I set about coming to terms with the difference between 'giving 100% effort when I practice' to 'practicing something 100% of the time'. Big difference. Giving 100% in effort means putting my heart and soul into what I choose to do when I choose to do it. The freedom I felt when I looked at it that way was massive. And then I got a little bit excited and wondered what practices should I choose?"

YOUR CONTRIBUTION

You know how sometimes you want to make a note in the margin of a book, and there's not quite enough room? Well, here's a little space to pop down a thought or two.

Need a nudge?

What are some words that come to mind after this chapter?

What activities have you attempted in the past, only to give up because you felt you weren't good enough, doing it enough?

What was the tripwire before? (Expectations of perfection? Lack of system? Lack of support? Not thoroughly defining the practice?)

Will you commit the time to thinking about your selections (and honing them) before you choose your practices?

Excellent! Now you can pull away from the station and begin your journey to your desired destination. Any thoughts or doodles?

*"Listen to your heart
before you speak.
Take a breath
before you write.
Pay yourself
before you spend.
Go again one more
time when you
want to quit.
Live each day
with passion."*

Kim White ★ 5 Guidelines For Life

Three

HOW WILL YOU BENEFIT?
LET US COUNT THE WAYS

This is what happens when you create real change within, by choosing 'when' freely, and regularly tracking your practices in 201 Day Achievement Principle:

☆ Your self-worth will expand because you experience a
  feeling of accomplishing something you have set your mind
  to. Rarely will you question your value or enough-ness.

☆ You will experience a newness, a freedom from

fear, because you've changed your relationship with achievement. You'll essentially shatter an 'all or nothing' paradigm, and in doing so you'll feel free, even when you are within a clock-schedule.

☆ You'll feel a sense of power because you've tapped into your own fuel source—choice.

☆ You'll take yourself seriously—as in for real—because you have proven that you can choose and then execute something important to you (essentially achieving worthiness through a manageable and doable self-accountability).

☆ You will not undervalue yourself, nor let your thoughts bully you, because you realize you're in charge.

☆ You will realize you can achieve anything because your mindset has shifted to one of proactivity blended with freedom.

☆ Daily, you'll feel expansive, energized, and excited.

☆ You will have an accelerated sense of fun and aliveness, and entertain ideas for future practices.

☆ You will—all of a sudden—see the immense power you have, and realize that the process of the 201 Day Achievement Principle is the tool with which to unleash it.

☆ Clarity, ease, and joy will come easily to you as a result of knowing you are always in charge.

Now it's your turn. How would I like to benefit?

"Fear loves generalization, and thrives on collecting in non-specific layers in the self. When you ask your fear to explain itself, much of it will emerge as smoke. Get specific with your 'fear' and much of it will disappear."

Teresa Easler

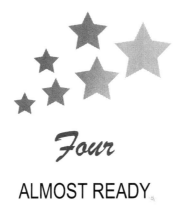

Four

ALMOST READY

Practices are chosen by amazing people with open minds—like you.

Practices are chosen by taking the time to consider all the angles around desired outcomes.

Practices, beyond all analysis, originate from a want that resides deep in the heart.

WHAT LIVES IN YOUR HEART?

What are some things that people say you are good at? Which ones do you believe?

What have been some of the things in the past that you've expressed interest in? Which ones have stayed with you?

Do any of these 'things' (that people say you're good at, that you believe you are good at, and/or in which you've expressed interest, and/or have stayed with you), appeal to you as a practice. What are they?

DREAM ONWARD

What is your dream job?

What does your perfect day look like?

Are there any 'things' in that job or in that day that you would consider choosing as a practice? What are they?

DREAM UPWARD

What is something you've always wanted to do but that scares you a little bit?

What is something you've always wanted to do that warms your heart?

What is something new in your world that you'd like to try?

AWAKEN

Of all the things that have crossed your mind since you started reading this book, what 'thing' or 'things' make you smile?

Of all the imaginings you've done since you started reading this book, what 'thing' keeps coming back to you over and over—no matter how unrealistic your 'reality' tells you it is—that 'thing' that just stays there and will not let go?

What would you choose if you were simply to abandon all thoughts of 'I don't know if I can do it for 201 days out of 365' and just adventure into it?

"Make your actions worthy to inspire others to dream more, learn more, and do more. Leadership is your actions not your title."

Kim White

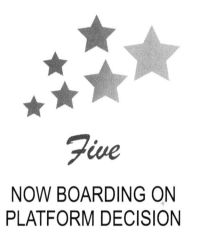

Five

NOW BOARDING ON
PLATFORM DECISION

GETTING UNSTUCK
LITTLE INSPIRATIONS
JOGGING YOUR MIND
PLANTING SEEDS

THE COMMON, THE UNCOMMON, THE WILD:
IF IT'S YOUR TRUE DESIRE THEN IT'S WONDER-FULL

1.   be an active participant in my neighbourhood

2.   put my clothes away – tidy bedroom

3.   wipe down/squeegee the shower after use

4.   eliminate coffee for the whole day / eliminate coffee before noon / after noon

5.   create (on paper/computer) a fantasy kingdom

6.   eat nothing after eight o'clock at night

7.   enjoy two servings of raw fruit a day

8.   enjoy two fresh veggies a day

9.   invent in my workshop

10.   send my adult children original and positive 'texts'

11.   write positive notes to my young children

12.   meditate once a day

13.   meditate twice a day

14.   move my body for more than fifteen minutes

15.   move my body for more than half an hour

16.   move my body for more than forty-five minutes

17.   move my body for an hour

18.   walk to work

19.   learn/practice a language

20. drink 10 glasses of water

21. eliminate pop/soda/soft drinks

22. eliminate flour

23. eliminate sugar

24. eliminate flour and sugar

25. avoid complaining

26. avoid swearing

27. compliment someone

28. recite a gratitude list before bed

29. write in my journal

30. read fiction

31. read nonfiction

32. read for pleasure

33. listen to music

34. send loving and positive thoughts to someone

35. write myself a love note

36. focus on three things I love about myself

37. compliment myself

38. work on my memoir

39. eat in

40. pray

41. tend my garden or houseplants

42. visit with my young children

43. read/storytell to my children

44. work on family tree/genealogy

45. write love letters to the world

46. create positive memes and share

47. abstain from news-cycle

48. immerse self in nature—city or country

49. celebrate my inner-child/my little self

50. spend time on ongoing 'clutter-clearing my home'

51. research travel destinations

52. record my spending

53. practice yoga

54. walk

55. run

56. treadmill

57. cook

58. make and consume elixirs

59. eat raw

60. abstain from meat

61. abstain from dairy

62. eat vegan

63. eat vegetarian

64. conversation with partner/spouse

65. delete email history to keep on top of it

66. consciously respond instead of reacting

67. regular moisturizing the body for self-care

68. longer showers for self-care and relaxation

69. outdoor time with my dogs

70. ride the bus to work

71. skateboard

72. bike to work

73. sketch and draw / learn / just do

74. paint/study painting

75. abstain from beer

76. calligraphy/studying calligraphy

77. sew

78. take photos

79. learn about my camera

80. do the dishes to keep my kitchen pretty

81. make the bed

82. pottery study or practice

83. dance naked each morning in my bedroom

84. do a 'morning bliss' ritual (comprised of specific practices)

85. do a nighttime wind-down routine (comprised of specific practices)

86. meet a set of daily standards (eg: drink water/converse with spouse/move my body)

87. nothing time – to sit and simply appreciate my surroundings

88. write poetry

89. learn to type/keyboard

90. crochet

91. knit

92. weave

93. embroider

94. cross stitch

95. plank for core strength

96. skip

97. carpentry / carve / whittle

98. have a go at soap making and creating bath bombs (could I have a spa business?)

99. history study

100. geography study

101. check in with my parent(s)

102. overview all careers (to be better informed of choices)

103. take action toward self-employment

104. compliment someone

105. belly laugh—exposure to comedy

106. swim

107. check on elderly neighbour

108. daydream and fantasize

109. mini-spa my life

110. learn basic home maintenance and repair

111. babysit for extra money toward a goal

112. trade childcare for me time

113. indulge in Netflix

114. make maps of fantasy worlds

115. create sci-fi realms

116. play chess

117. learn chess

118. read a set of identified classics (literature)

119. practice stand-up comedy

120. juggle

121. perform/rehearse stage role (with a view to future auditions)

122. sing hymns

123. renovate that room/basement/garage that's been wanting a redo

124. make something from nothing

125. add to recording my family story

126. sort photos (electronic and other)

127. collage

128. mural a wall

129. listen to motivating podcasts

130. research true crime

131. work on any of my practices at my fave café – go off location

132. create and worship at a home altar/shrine/sanctuary space

133. take a different route home

134. get up an hour earlier

135. go to bed an hour earlier

136. do lunch at a different time

137. try different/new foods

138. establish conversations with the self

139. create my own meditations

140. support others

141. engage with an online group that supports me

142. attend AA in person

143. attend NA in person

144. have lunch away from the computer/electronics

145. eat mindfully—focus on tasting the food and considering its origins

146. abstain from electronics in bedroom

147. ask a loved one/friend/family about his or her dreams

148. show increased interest and focus on a randomly chosen activity/project that is part of the day

149. listen wholeheartedly

150. establish silent times with no speaking and no background noise

151. have an 'English' tea break

152. eat cacao – through heirloom chocolate (and other superfoods)

153. learn to craft chocolate

154. forage – or learn/read about foraging

155. get outside the house for any reason

156. open a window and let the air in

157. communicate with someone by fb, email, or phone

158. stand outside, barefooted if possible, and feel the ground

159. night-sky or day-sky gaze

160. experience the sunrise/be up and present for it

161. do 'in front of mirror' affirmations

162. dress in clothing that reflects the true me

163. do something different with my hair

164. go makeup free

165. visit the gym

166. avoid television/streaming shows/movies

167. take time to go inside myself and visit my future self for direction

168. participate in making the world a better place

169. consciously put goodness into the world in random ways

170. consciously seek and locate goodness in the world and acknowledge it

171. reupholster a piece of furniture

172. puzzle time: jigsaw/crossword

173. light a candle

174. savour a particular coffee I enjoy (and/or discover more)

175. take the time to be conscious of myself in a moment / example: learn to watch myself do something

176. read about spiritual leaders

177. bathe/tub

178. mind my own business/abstain from gossip

179. collect, tag, and store items for annual garage sale

180. remove one significant item from my home (recycle, donate, trash)

181. sit on my comfortable sofa that's meant for sitting

182. job shadow/volunteer in the field I want to work in

183. upgrade my skills in an area I know I want to pursue/work in

184. establish myself with a theatre company as a stage-hand/ helper and get regular shifts

185. bring joy to 'the table' wherever I go: smile, interact, draw happy faces, round-up for tips, open doors

186. drive without road rage

187. create a podcast about my speciality

188. live in the moment – be spontaneous – trust my gut

189. learn Morse Code

190. discover orienteering (read/participate)

191. become active in an environmental group

192. embrace activism

193. kayak (learn, read about, save for a kayak, purchase, lessons) over a year

194. become a clown (self-taught, lessons, clown school, costuming)

195. down-time: regular, random acts of self-indulgence involving laughter and kindness

196. martial arts

197. release tension and upcycle thoughts session

198. give up watching sports in favour of family activities

199. cycling

200. join a sports team

201. choose a course at a local technical college/finish it/homework

**USE THIS SPACE TO ELABORATE ON
ANY OR MANY OF THE ABOVE**

"Passion is at the core of all communication. Where is your heart?"

Teresa Easler

Six

CATEGORIES

You're all prepped and ready to choose. Should you share your choices right away with others? Double check that your choices are realistic? Get a shot of confidence from a friend or, alternatively, possibly a little criticism and even a 'You're doing what?' (From the naysayer in the family.) Should you share before? After? At all?

Whether you are aware of this or not, you are the expert of you. Ultimately, you make the choices for your practices, the decisions around how and when to track, where to keep your tracking journal—or whether you'll use the app—and even who you are going to share your plans with.

If you've been an active participant in this book, you will be well prepared.

Perhaps you have already joined the Facebook group to see what other people have done.

It comes down to this: this is not 'the rest of your life', it is a *part* of the rest of your life. But, it is an important part of your life, as it may well be a corner you're turning or a crossroads from which you are moving on. Your practice may well lead to a new business, a promotion, or another kind of growth that will benefit you in myriad ways.

The intentions of this handbook that companions the tracking journal is to emphasize that 201 Day Achievement Principle is not a fad. It is a way of life. A style of growth.

Your choice is not a means to an end, it is a means to a start.

☆ Choose mindfully.

☆ Choose only practices you want, that you covet, that you desire.

☆ Choose now... or almost right now. Read the rest of the book, and then choose. Sooner than later. (Note: later is like a taxi called on New Year's Eve—it never arrives.)

☆ Choose however many practices you feel comfortable with. Many people like the number 'three'. If you're going to 'subgroup', then you might end up with more because you are 'niching' or categorizing (remember the dairy example?)

A Means To A Start

Pilot group member, Camille, had the 'means to a start' in mind when she chose three practices. Her first choice was something she knew she was already fairly strong at. Something she knew would be doable. She wanted to make sure to have something that she wanted, and for which an already proven dedication would serve to cheer her on.

Her second choice was something she wanted that she was a little 'shaky' on. She called this a nudge.

For the third practice, she chose something that she wanted but was not doing at all. Something she knew would be a challenge.

"The way I chose, graduating the level of challenge for myself, was a way of holding my own hand." *Camille A.*

Niched And Unleashed

Just as business has specialists—niche markets catering to specific needs—you can niche practice. The results are sure to inform you what part of a practice you are stronger at.

'Jerry Example' knows he wants to abstain from sugar and flour for 201 out of 365 days. He can put that as one practice, or he can separate and have sugar as one and flour as another. The benefit of this is that he'll be able to see, in short order, which of the two he's most heavily reliant upon. And, he won't feel like he messed up if he hits his target on flour but not on sugar. One will not affect the other.

'Evelyn Case-in-Point' is wanting to write a book. She totally gets the logic behind 201 days out of 365. Evelyn knows that there are a lot of aspects to writing a book. She could lump them all into one practice she calls 'the book', or she can separate the components into 'reading books on writing' and 'composing the manuscript'.

Words Matter

Next comes what you will name your practice. We're not kidding. It's important. For Evelyn to see the 'title of her book' in her tracking journal will be much more motivating and inspiring than seeing the word 'writing' or 'working on my book'. Niched and unleashed she might choose: MY LIBRARY, AUTHOR'S CORNER, or LOOK OUT HEMINGWAY.

Likewise, imagine how Jerry will feel seeing HEALTHY ME instead of 'no sugar'. If Jerry lets creativity run wild he might even end up with SWEET ME and FLOUR POWER.

Words really mattered to our journal designer, Theresa M.

One of her practices was to exercise.

Several weeks into her practice of exercise and she wasn't feeling it. When she examined why she felt exercise was an obstacle, she realized that the word was off-putting for her. She had never thought of herself as athletic, and she associated the word exercise with athletics. Theresa is perceptive; creativity is her career. She reframed her choice, and called it MOVEMENT, then she further honed it to MORE PLAY.

Immediately, she felt the shift. In short order, she was outside playing with her children, making snowmen, pulling the sled, even shoveling snow —all exercise if you hadn't noticed. The word exercise had negative connotations for her. Play made her smile. Her participation went up.

The point is, if you begin with a creative high, then you are essentially piling on the positive at the front end. While this is going to be a year, starting from the day you launch, you can modify your 'titles' as you learn about yourself. And there will be other years to modify.

If you're really eager and things are going swimmingly, there can even be new practices started within the year which operate on their own yearly cycle. You may find that six months into your launch, while you are moving along with the three practices you chose, you notice that your energy has been low midmorning. As you acknowledge you never eat breakfast, you might decide this is the perfect opportunity to take what you've learned about choosing and tracking, and start a new year for that one new practice of 'eating breakfast' (HAPPY MORNING BELLY) 201 out of 365 days a year. At that point, you already know how to track. You've already seen the benefits. Evaluate if it will overwhelm and, if it will not, then go for it.

How Many Should I Choose?

The best way to decide how many practices to choose is to see how many are on your list and, if there are more than a few, then begin eliminating those which are not as high a priority. All on that list should be wants not shoulds, so you'll be eliminating based on what those practices will bring to your life—and the fun factor.

You may be super-excited, but you do not need to be super-overwhelmed. And there's nothing to say you might not touch on some of the things that are not selected, regardless of tracking. And there's no stopping you from tracking those things in six or nine months' time. If your list is two things, consider digging deep to mine the depths of your 'wanting'. Sometimes we don't go far enough because we are fearful the choice will seem 'silly', or not be a 'real thing'. All wants are real and lead to real somethings. Let no one write your script for you.

That's one reason why we did the 201 choices page—not to make you choose something obscure, but to validate the creative and the wild, and to show that they are as meaningful as the conventional choices (exercise, healthy eating).

Sometimes the more wild, the more wonderful. The more you stretch, the more you change. The more you change, the more adventure in your life. Lookout career #2, watch out totally unexpected life-direction. Yes! Now you get the idea. Pull the socks up on that crazy 'want' and bring it onto the page. Sheesh, even if your tracking shows a low number at the end of the year (for that choice), it will still be way more than you would have done had you not entertained that practice at all. Nothing is ever lost when your numbers for a choice are low. It's like market analysis on yourself; you'll discover how important something really is.

TAKEAWAYS

★ Invite the wonder-filled choices.

★ Eliminate any sneaky shoulds.

★ Niche and unleash.

★ Name your practices.

FAQ

If I choose to split my practice up into several categories, will there be room? What if I did that and then still had more practices?
Our tracking journal has seven spots for you to write your practices. The earlier dairy example (splitting into four) was an extreme, yet it is also advisable for someone who truly wants to learn from their tracking and maintain a high degree of motivation. If you split one of your practices into four, you'd still have three more spaces for other practices. And remember, we recommend starting with three practices—don't overwhelm yourself.

ANOTHER BIT OF EAVESDROPPING
INTERJECTION/EXCERPT:
A PARTICIPANT SHARES

"I wanted so much. I wanted to increase my knowledge for every fricking topic I'd ever found interesting. I wanted to super-size my choices. That's how pumped I was. But, as I settled down and read more of the book, I started to feel more like the tortoise than the hare—in a good way. When I analyzed what was realistic in my life, I narrowed my choices. I told myself, there is always next year. If I choose ten, and I burn out on all, there might not be a next year. I channeled the wise tortoise. I told myself it didn't mean I'd never learn calligraphy. When I reduced my list, I noticed that I leaned toward lifestyle choices such as exercise and eating. I had long wanted to make sure I was eating healthier foods—and it wasn't a should, I truly love fresh veggies and fruit—and I also knew I used to love it when I cycled, so that wasn't a should either. I went with those two. Then I added upgrading my math, because I want to be more confident at work when we do measure-ups for flooring. Then I thought to myself that there also needed to be an additional element of fun; that while I wanted growth in 'health' and in 'academics' I also wanted FUN. (Not that I couldn't be creative with my other choices and make them fun). So I decided on one more practice and chose something off the charts for me but that had long intrigued me: juggling. I had four. And it felt great."

THE FLOOR IS YOURS – YOUR SPACE

You've come a long way through this book and taken in a lot of information. What is the most important thing you've learned so far about the topic of tracking, our project, and yourself?

"When you realize that choice equals freedom, you will discover what you've been preparing for your whole life."

Teresa Easler

Seven

BALLOONS AND STREAMERS
- MAKE SOME NOISE

The Importance Of Celebration

Take a photo or two or ten. A selfie with your tracking journal. Pose
with this book. Grab your bike, knitting needles, French phrase
book, shovel and seeds, welding rod, or prayer beads—essentially
whatever represents your practice. Even record a quick video. Make
sure to pump your arm a few times. You're on your way.

Milestones, like first day of school, birthdays, anniversaries, mortgage burnings, represent growth. That's why milestones are treasured. They are what marks time when shaping life. And that is why it's great to celebrate them. Each celebration marks a timeframe, be it a month or a decade of experience, a stretch of strength, a measure of accomplishment. When people take the time to celebrate these markers, that recognition is reflected in their health—physical and mental. Collectively, the milestone and celebration builds a healthy self-concept.

Physical Self

Celebrating is good for all of us, whether we're the guest or the person celebrating. Get-togethers are opportunities for conversation and laughter, even movement and activity. Who hasn't enjoyed a night 'glow-bowling' with a group of friends to mark some milestone? There's a level of anticipation and excitement when there's some kind of recognition planned. When we celebrate an achievement, we inspire others. When any of us attend and celebrate with someone who has achieved, we are inspired. It's all about growth and feeling good.

Mental Health

That growth and feeling good translates to being sociable and its benefits. When any of us connect with others we tell stories and feel close to people, regardless of whether they are new or besties. There is strength when there are supportive people, and there is a transference of positive energy when people share and celebrate what is meaningful in life.

View Of Self

Taking the time to celebrate milestones is a fantastic way to self-nurture. Whether you are alone, with a small group, or throwing a big get-together, celebration is a way to say to yourself that you matter. Yes, even a selfie and a comment can do that. Even a coffee at a local spot can be self-nurturing. Celebrating a milestone, and enjoying and marking the smaller steps that lead up to that milestone, is a way to show yourself that you matter.

When you start your practice: celebrate. Build in windows for your unique way of celebrating, and, by all means, regardless of what percentage you hit at 365, ensure you do a year end.

The Launch

Planning Your Launch - It's A Big Deal

☆ Coffee date with a few friends where you show them the books and tell them your choices.

☆ Flowers (picked or purchased) for yourself.

☆ The purchase of a potted plant which will remind you of your ongoing growth and need to nurture.

☆ A one year subscription to a magazine or YouTube channel that will remind you of your own 365.

☆ A well-crafted, celebratory-mood email to your closest friends and family, announcing the start of a new year.

☆ Dinner with yourself at a fine restaurant.

☆ Cupcakes and candles with your family.

☆ A post and a symbolic photo on the 201 Day Achievement Principle Facebook page.

☆ The first of a monthly social media post that shares a positivity (of growth) message.

☆ Mirror time—you in front of your mirror—introducing the new you (as if you were at a job for the first day), stating your strengths, and smiling.

☆ Create 31 positive messages, relating to your choices, on cards or pieces of paper, put them into a container, and place them beside your bathroom sink, so that you can pull one a day and read it in the morning. When all the days in the month have been pulled, they go back into the container for the next month.

☆ If you have the cash and freezer space, 12 bags of a favourite, decadent fruit (blackberries?) so that on your monthaversary you pull them out and enjoy.

☆ A complete day out at a park, botanical garden, museum, library, mall to celebrate you.

☆ A makeover—haircut and style.

☆ A cleansing of your home.

☆ A crazy dance to mark the beginning of a projected monumental year.

☆ Prayer.

☆ A glass of wine with a heartfelt toast.

☆ Sleep under the stars—or stay up late and sit under the stars.

☆ A pot luck with your closest friends.

☆ A donation to a charity close to your heart.

The Day You Start

Whether you choose a simple and sacred way to mark the beginning, or you blow up balloons and have a party for one at your house or at a favourite spot, make it memorable. Treat it with reverence. Give and gift yourself this 'date' and this beginning. You. Are. Worth. It.

Know you may feel a bit jittery. You may have moments where you doubt yourself before you have even started. Remind yourself that this is different. There is no one expecting a streak—100% commitment.

The essential yes/no guide to your launch day:

Symbolic?: yes
Expensive?: no

Celebratory?: yes
Shame or Scarcity based?: no

Enthusiasm?: yes
Apathy?: no

Ceremonial?: yes
Sacrificial?: no

This time next year you will be well practiced. What might this day next year look like?

HAVING THE TIME OF YOUR LIFE

Ten pounds lighter
Ten-fold stronger
Tenth grade finished
Ten chapters written

Increased energy
Increased interest
Increased awareness
Increased ability

More confidence
More money
More friends
More marketable skills

Extra behemoth volume completely read
Excellence in participation in class and a fluency in French
Enthusiastically complete—your manuscript in rough draft
End of project: a sweater knit

TAKEAWAYS

- ★ Make it a big deal.

- ★ Monthaversary it on your calendar.

- ★ Treat it as a life event worthy of the word
  milestone—not just 'another' program.

FAQ

Too shy, too private, too quiet to share. I keep myself to myself. How can I benefit from celebration when I am a loner?
With deep respect to your need, comfort, and choice to be private, let us make the point that, ultimately, the person who needs inviting to the ball is you. A selfie can be taken but need not be shared. A candle or two or ten is still appropriate—you can light them and blow them out in the company of you. You recognizing you is the most important thing of all. Quite a few of the points on the list of ideas are suited to individual celebration. Whatever you choose to do, make sure to shout out your praises for yourself. And, if you like, send us a private email. We'd love to celebrate your journey and we promise to keep your information private.

LISTENING TO THE THOUGHTS OF OTHERS
INTERJECTION/EXCERPT:
A PARTICIPANT SHARES

"I don't have tons of cash to throw a party. But something did feel 'celebratory' about ushering in this new me. I hadn't realized how important it was to 'make this a big deal'. Once I read the list and the explanation—especially the mental health part—I began to ask myself why not? Why not post a selfie on the Facebook group—one saying I had just chosen four practices. When I did, and saw the people there, I realized that 201 Day Achievement Principle is different than other 'programs'; far beyond the amazing way it allows for so much freedom in the target, in the 201 days out of 365. It shows how we can honour ourselves wherever we are in our journey. A few days after I posted I looked back at the list of suggestions and I decided that I would make myself a card, like a birthday card, but with the word CELEBRATE written on the front, and a 'you're one your way' message inside. I put it on my desk. Just seeing it there reminded me that I have started to realize how 'worthy' I am, and how cool the practices I've chosen are. The making of the card, the putting it on my desk, and the tucking it in the back of the journal to bring it out at another time, was super-powerful. I might even make myself another card in a month or so. A congratulations card with a 'great going so far' inside it."

SPACE TO STRETCH YOUR THOUGHTS

PART II

Tracking

"Never let anything you want make you forget what you have. It is what you already have that is the foundation to get what you want."

Kim White

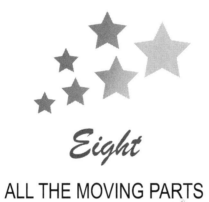

Eight

ALL THE MOVING PARTS

PART I covered choosing a practice. PART II covers the system of tracking the practice.

In a perfect world, choosing and tracking, should never be separated. And it's not just something we made up.

Before his retirement in 1933, British mathematician and statistician, Karl Pearson stated: *"When performance is measured, performance improves. When performance is measured and reported back, the rate of improvement accelerates."* Thereafter it became known as Pearson's Law.

The correlation between recording participation and success has been lauded by universities and business development types from all walks of life. Stand by for some massive studies.

Tracking And You

Tracking is a way to learn about yourself. It's a statement of 'time and care for the self'. It's a gesture of prioritizing you and your future. And, because of its impact, it can be said that tracking is a kind of practice of its own.

Choosing a practice, then tracking when you do it and when you don't do it, is the finest service you'll ever perform for yourself.

Call it abbreviated journaling.
You are creating a record.
A record of you.
And that is meaningful.
A contract between you and you.
You become your own biggest fan—not in a
'look at me' way, but in a 'look in me' way.

In 201 Day Achievement Principle a 'yes, I did it' or 'no, I didn't do it'—however you decide to mark it (a check mark or X, a Y or N, a happy face or slash)—are each a measure of success because each indicate that the act of tracking took place. Recording or tracking is productive.

The target is 201 days out of 365. 201 / 365 = 55%. Aiming to do something 55% of the time, 201 days out of 365, is a fantastic intention because it:

☆ Prevents burnout.

☆ Promotes a healthy sense of self-acceptance.

☆ Advocates realistic balance.

☆ Encourages adding more practices (which supports personal growth).

And because it is unrealistic to have an unbroken streak of participation in any practice, and beyond stressful to maintain any uber-high percentage, we believe that:

55% is the new 100%.

Realistic participation basically guarantees consistent participation which equates to an end of the year practice that has generated success. Put simply, it's a sweater knit, a language learned, a trilogy read, a novel written, a weight-loss realized, a fitness goal met, three balls juggled. Whatever your 'want'—the desire that became a practice—clarity in choice and realistic expectation of participation will get you a successful outcome. Essentially, 55% is flipping-fantastic.

Whether you 'do' something and track it or 'do not do' something and track it, tracking is powerful. However you record—checkmark, X, star, happy face—your 'I didn't do it' is a shout out to freedom. And that's the beauty of 201 Day Achievement Principle.

YOUR 'no' is a shout-out to FREEDOM.

We repeat: to track is to learn about yourself. If you end up with zero after the first few weeks, there may be a valid reason (not excuse): you could have fallen ill, or you may have chosen something you thought you should choose versus what you wanted to choose.

**201 Day Achievement Principle marries tracking
with a chosen practice to result in your success.
No matter what percentage you hit, it's
a win as long as you tracked it.**

The system, over time, builds your foundation of consistency; it hones your heart to select the practices that most benefit you. And that is something that no other 'system' or program does.

NOTE: Do not mistake results under 55% for laziness. Any participation is a win because, as long as you are practicing tracking, you are winning (learning, thinking, and participating).

Competitive attitudes and focus on streaks (all or nothing) will result in measuring yourself against some kind of 'invisible competitor'. This will bring about an 'end' (because all streaks end), which will bring on guilt, which will create excuses to not begin again.

201 Day Achievement Principle supports stops and starts within its framework. You simply continue 'to do' or 'not do' something based on the choice that you have committed to for a year.

A Little Science, A Little High

To be motivated is to get closer to success. So what creates motivation? Well, it turns out that when people register a win, a little triumph, or an accomplishment, the brain releases dopamine. Dopamine is connected to the feeling of pleasure. When each of us experiences pleasure, we tend to want to repeat it.

Checking off items—any of those lists, calendars, or journals of the 'I did this practice today' variety, delivers a little dopamine. If those items on the list are clear, doable, and quick to accomplish: Hello Motivation!

People need to experience only a small success in order to generate motivation. Once the cycle of success is entered, the formula kicks in: little success = motivation = more success = greater motivation (and so on). It's pretty much unstoppable.

So, the secret to maintaining motivation is to ensure you set yourself up for success in increments. Many of us know this as breaking a project into pieces and celebrating each of the parts or pieces along the way to total completion. Generating motivation from achieving mini goals within a major goal is a much better way to go than waiting until the end of a project to 'feel' and 'celebrate' any sense of achievement.

Neuroscientists call the eagerness to repeat actions as 'self-directed learning'. The more eager people are, the more likely they'll achieve what it is they wanted, be it learning a language, renovating a house, playing an instrument competently, writing a book, or becoming physically fit enough to run a marathon.

We've created the winning formula for you to succeed. It begins with identifying and being clear about what you truly want. Next comes understanding the difference between practice and habit, and the freedom attached to choosing 'to do' or 'not to do' your practice. After that, the winning formula is completed by recording your participation. This system of success opens the door for a dopamine delivery. This generates pleasure, which creates motivation—leading you to accomplish your goals.

Creating a visual—having a tangible reminder of your wants along with your tracking system—is huge. The important part is that the tracking needs to be as simple as possible—a short and not too time-consuming exercise. Enough to record and receive the dose of dopamine, but not so cumbersome that the tracking itself becomes a chore.

Don't Just Take Our Word For It

The American Psychological Association summarized a long report in October 2015:

"If you are trying to achieve a goal, the more often that you monitor your progress, the greater the likelihood that you will succeed, according to research. Your chances of success are even more likely if you report your progress publicly or physically record it."

Lead author, Benjamin Harkin, PhD, University of Sheffield, concurred in the journal *Psychological Bulletin*, saying that the

APA's review suggested that prompting 'progress monitoring' did improve behavioural performance, and therefore increased the likelihood of reaching one's goals.

Harkin and his colleagues conducted a meta-analysis of 138 studies comprising 19,951 participants. They set about looking at the effectiveness of an 'intervention' or a 'treatment' designed to prompt participants into monitoring/recording their goal progress. The goals noted were mainly personal health goals like weight loss, lowering blood pressure, or quitting smoking. They found that the prompts to monitor increased the success of the participants. And the more frequent the 'monitoring', the greater the success.

This is significant, since the meta study was comprised of almost 20,000 participants. Harkin said: "Prompting people to monitor their progress can help them to achieve their goals, but some methods of monitoring are better than others. Specifically, we would recommend that people be encouraged to record, report or make public what they find out as they assess their progress."

This supports the informal information from our pilot group who used 201 Day Achievement tracking journals—which are likely much more user-friendly than those used in scientific studies.

There's more: not only has the success of tracking—recording participation—been proven by the 201 Day Achievement Principle originators, but the 55% is notable in that it appears in the range of another recent study by a small personal growth firm, Precision Nutrition, which went as far as to calculate a participation range for success. They noted that the most successful participants in their program were those who 'practiced' between 50 and 79% of the time. In other words, those participants who engaged in a particular activity more than 80% of the time found it difficult to keep that up—ultimately unable to reach their goal. Likewise, motivation was lost and practice fell off when their participants engaged in the activity less than 50% of the time—not that they weren't getting some value.

In PN's study, the sweet spot was 50-79%. It fits perfectly with our findings of 55%.

More On Recording

Counting without a written record is only good until a person forgets. Take running laps in a gymnasium or on an oval: how many was that? Unless someone is using a clicker, it's hard to keep count.

A few times a week is not an exact number.

Tracking what you do, be it with a full-on sentence of touchy-feely feedback, or a Y or N, will allow you to release the need to mentally track, and it will create an accurate record.

Was it 3 or 4 times? It might have only been 2 because I had that appointment.

Well, if it was 4 times that's great, and if it was 2 times that's fine as well, but 2 is half of 4. Do you not want accuracy? It's nice to know. That's the purpose of 201 Day Achievement Principle. We want you to know your true input and participation.

In reality, guessing is the gentler cousin of outright untruth. Every one of us is worthy of the truth. When people are honest with themselves they grow in character. Tracking removes all guesswork.

Your choice of practice, the freedom of choice to do it or not to do it based on targeting 201 out of 365 days, and your accuracy of tracking your participation, is connected—it's all one collective success-building exercise.

Make Your Mark

It's a checkmark, an X, a Y for yes, or whatever symbol you decide. A happy face, your initials, a star. Maybe, as in a few of our participants, it's the actual running calculation (more on the simple math later)—the actual numbers within the square allotted for each day.

When you make your mark, you create an indelible print image that signals your successful personal 'brand'. Never underestimate the power of tracking.

TAKEAWAYS

- ★ If you are willing to track, then you are willing to grow.
- ★ Choice + Tracking = Goals Realized.
- ★ Streaks end, consistency wins.
- ★ Making your mark is literally life changing.
- ★ Make your mark your BRAND.

FAQ's

You talk about Y for yes and N for no, or whatever works best to record 'both doing and not doing' in the journal, but wouldn't a blank indicate a no? Why would I track a no? I could just count only the yeses and ignore the blanks.

This is true. The bonus of tracking all participation, whether it is a yes or a no, is that it gets us used to the power of tracking. Pen on the paper no matter what. Finger on the keyboard (for the app) no matter what. Not doing something, and then *not* writing down that we didn't do it, is quite different than not doing something and writing down that we did not do it. The latter has a bit of a super-power of 'urging' us to think again and go do it. Additionally, leaving a blank leaves doubt—did I forget to put a yes? Create your own system that supports your continued practice within the system we've created for you, but make sure to consider that the more exposure you have to your journal, the more your practice—and the reasons you chose it—will be on your mind.

Tell me again why, if I am less than 55%, it's still a win?
Because the very fact that you're tracking means you're paying attention to something that you decided was meaningful to you. You will be learning as long as you're tracking. Even if you tracked zero, you would learn that this practice was not important enough to you, or needed to be adjusted in the length of time you'd decided was a recordable 'yes' for a session. Any tracking informs. 55% has been proven to be in the sweet spot of achieving success. That doesn't mean less than 55% will lead nowhere. The very action of tracking, and arriving at say, 25%, shows you are doing something. Something is more than nothing. 'Nothing' is often the result of aiming high—as in all or nothing. If 25% feels 'slack' to you, compare it to having set an all or nothing goal for sugar consumption, and then having had wine on day three—alcohol contains sugar. You cave. Your absolute was just shattered. You start again. Three days later you are given a box of chocolates. Eventually, if you're like most people, your resolve will collapse. You will be upset with yourself for not 'sticking to your plan'. At the end of a few months, most likely a few weeks, you will forgo the goal. It feels impossible. You keep beating yourself up about it. So you stop. But if you had aimed for 201/365, and even if you ended up 25%, that is better than the zero you would have achieved from quitting an all or nothing target. No matter your number, at the end of a year you'll be much further ahead than the perfection route.

LISTENING IN ON THE THOUGHTS OF OTHERS
INTERJECTION/EXCERPT:
A PARTICIPANT SHARES

"I thought I'd remember to record my twenty-minutes of playing the piano but, by Friday, I couldn't pin down if I'd done it Sunday and Monday or just Monday. I didn't want to cheat and have the numbers be like a lie, but I felt ripped off by not putting in two days, so I decided that, either way, it would have been easier to keep the book handy and pop a checkmark in there. Better yet, even though I had other practices, keeping the book on the music stand made sense. The piano is in the centre of the house and I am always passing by it, so it'd be handy to record doing (or not doing) my other practices too."

A Little Space To Spread Out

If you've ever had to fill in a tracking or checklist before, how was that experience for you?

If you sense it will be overwhelming to track, what will help?

Is it helpful to know you can just put a check, you don't have to write a novel?

Do you have a classic 'doodle' or an original 'stickperson' that makes you smile? (Why not use that?) Judy uses hearts. Stars are common. What about the moon?

Think way back—do you have a favourite memory of when you received a 'star' or 'sticker' for something you did?

How did it make you feel?

"Your best teachers
are the ones who
pull the wisdom
out of you,
rather than
just telling you
what to do."

Kim White

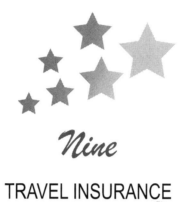

Nine

TRAVEL INSURANCE

We hear you saying: "I get the concept, now just tell me how to work out the percentage, and show me the journal."

We love that you're enthusiastic—ready to rock your own world. You've already got a fair amount of power behind you, and a lot of 'I wanna accomplish something' in your heart.

Whether you're itching to lock in your choices, or a little anxious that you might not choose wisely, there is more we'd like to share that others have gone through when they prepare and then endeavour on 201 Day Achievement Principle.

If we were your guardians, and you were going on an expedition across the Sahara, we'd want to make sure your plan was solid. It would be vital for us to supply a leak-proof water bottle.

We want to prepare you for what might happen on your 201 Day Achievement Principle journey.

We want to make sure you're fully prepared. That goes beyond understanding the basic concept and how to calculate your percentage. When you fully participate in 201 Day Achievement Principle, you will be set free from all the paradigms you've learned so far in life about accomplishing goals.

Despite all the talk about how the tracking itself is a sign of success—and the studies that back up that statement—some people are simply not used to writing in a journal. Some are electronic wizards and not used to being accountable on paper—fear not, there's an app.

Whether or not you use the app, it's important to know that, while it's speedy to click, there is a relationship formed between you and your goals when a few words are written. Even the value of a symbol—as mentioned before, your personal mark—is powerful. Many are those who have smiled after drawing a happy face.

Don't Knock It Until You've Tried It

If you've written in the space provided in this book, you might already have experienced the connection writing can offer between you and yourself. If you haven't used the space, we encourage you to give it a shot.

The pen is mightier than the sword.

There's a bond between the heart and the page, the soul and the ink.

Intentions take on superpowers when sketched or written.

Yes, it may take time to get used to. Prepare yourself by simply knowing that. Be open to change. We have it on good authority that, in a pinch, a decent record-keeping entry can be done for several practices in less than a minute. We also know that a sentence or two has generated the momentum for the next day's participation.

The main reason that tracking might seem to be time consuming is that you are simply not used to being so accountable. Consistency around practices—whether you do them or not—is substantiated, buoyed, and powered by entering the yes or no into the tracking journal, or the tracking app.

You may get carried away with the romance of the choices you've made, and generate all kinds of energy around the outcomes you want to see and, in that headiness, you can forget that the tracking is largely responsible for the successful result.

You may well encounter an internal struggle. "My excitement was there in the choosing. Not so much in the doing. I'm glad it's not one-hundred percent, but I'm struggling even to participate."

Know this: you are normal. This is change. Humans are not typically big on change. We're all human beings, but not all human doings. People get into patterns of doing 'stuff'. Even when—if analyzed—that 'stuff' slows them or holds them back.

Breaking through and making change includes making tracking convenient for yourself—it's the key to your success.

There's good reason we're rambling on about tracking: we want you to get really familiar with recording what you do. Ways to make tracking convenient include:

☆ Make the physical tracker visible so that you cannot ignore its presence. In sight, in mind.

☆ Ensure there's always a pen right beside the tracker.

☆ Link tracking with a routine that is a given—like going to bed.

Another 'normal' is, "I never keep things up—this is how I am, so this is how I'll always be."

Where would you be without preconceived notions? Probably a lot further than you are. Well, now's your time to find out. Imagine if you never took a step forward, sideways, or backward. You'd stay in exactly the same place. You'd atrophy. You'd starve. Sure, this is extreme, but think about it: you don't stay in the same place. You move around, you go and make your lunch, you walk over to a friend's, you go on road trips. Each of those things began with a thought and an action. Over time you've changed some of those actions. You've gone on different road trips, you've made different lunches, you've gained new friends and dropped others. You have changed.

Humans are not only a work of art, they are a work in progress, and are ever-changing. From the ongoing replication of cells to tastes and likes and dislikes, people may be averse to change, but they move—or are carried away—with the times nonetheless.

If you recognize that you might throw things in your own way, awareness is a good thing, because you can be prepared with solutions.

The things you might trip yourself with include mental blocks and the physical ones associated with tracking. We know the journal is not heavy or bulky, but there are people who might find it an issue to tote around. Ask yourself what else you carry around and if there is room for the tracker. Find yourself a logical, physical place in your home where you are sure to 'check in' or visit daily. Some people use the bedside table for end-of-the-day recording. This makes a lot of sense because the end of the day is when you have likely accomplished, or not, your practices. It's also a time when you still remember what you did. It's that 'interval' when you likely have nothing else left to do but check in with self.

Anecdotal Pause: Combining Recording With An Existing Ritual

Team member, Natalie, reads before she goes to bed. It's something she does every night, and always has. She says that it's part of her nighttime routine. When she began tracking her practices she found that the tracking journal was often in a different place—where she had left it last. A busy mom with a gazillion things to do, she decided that she'd put the tracking journal on her bedside table with her current read. It was an instant win. It was easy to record her practices right before she read each night.

Support

Some folks really thrive with an accountability partner. Partners come in various forms. Take the Facebook page, for example. There's a powerful presence on our page. Determination and positivity abound. The Facebook page is a sure place to find someone who has a practice that is similar or even the same as yours. It's a spot to locate a likeminded match. It's also a place to see the practices of others and be inspired by them. Many a friendship has been made through social media, and our Facebook page *201 Day Achievement Principle* is a perfect place to connect. We can't think of a better location to inspire someone, or be inspired, or both.

The solution to obstacles is largely anticipation, and then a huge dose of objectivity. And the ability to reframe.

TAKEAWAYS

★ We can change. We're renewing all the time.

★ The Scouts are right: be prepared.

★ In sight, in mind.

FAQ

What is your Facebook page called again? Do I have to be approved or can I just join in?

We are under the banner of 201 Day Achievement Principle. Find us and click to be added. You can also Join us on Instagram @201DayAchievementPrinciple, or feel free to send us direct messages through:

201dayachievementprinciple@connecttothecore.com

LISTENING IN ON THE THOUGHTS OF OTHERS
INTERJECTION/EXCERPT:
A PARTICIPANT SHARES

"At first I thought it was overkill to have a book all about how to choose and how to track. Why not give me a page of instructions and the journal and let me at it? But I realize tracking is more than just a checkmark (even if I did choose to use a checkmark). It's totally connected to the choosing. The two are inseparable. They make a process. A growth process. It's my time, it's my development, and it's my growth. I'm worth all the consideration, rather than a quick decision of 'okay here are some things I've sucked at before, and I think I should be better at.' No. It's more than that. It's personal development. It's time well spent thinking about how I'm going to become a better performer at some new stuff or some old stuff. It's all important stuff. Including being ready for any obstacles, and especially reminding myself that the very nature of being a human means I am changing. I never realized how cool it would feel to create my own mark—a brand. My own brand. I went back over the pages and filled in some of the questions that I really hadn't thought important when I first started reading."

HOW'S IT GOING?

How do you feel you might respond to keeping up with the tracking?

What benefits would you find in an app?

What benefits would you find in the paper-pen method?

Which way do you lean? Are you willing to give pen and paper a try?

How do you feel about it all so far?

"Be the leader of your life. You have total control of your 'choices'."

Teresa Easler

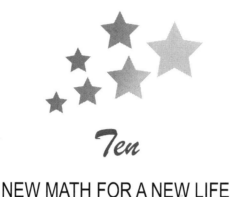

Ten

NEW MATH FOR A NEW LIFE

We know that 201 days out of a year (365 days) is 55%. More than half the year. Here's a quick guide: 4 days a week is 57%. Of course, this is not a weekly program. This is a full year in which you can calculate your percentage at any time to know how you are currently doing in your quest to hit 55% for the year.

Tracking your progress at any time during YOUR year

Let's make this simple. Please follow along on your calculator:

A   How many days since you started?

B   How many days have you practiced?

C   Take your number of days practiced (B) and divide by (A) the number of days since you started.

D   On your calculator this will show you a decimal point and a 'number'.

E   Remove the decimal before the number and place a percentage sign after the first two numbers.

Example

A   14 days (I started 14 days ago)

B   10 days (I have practiced – tracked YES in the journal)

C   10 divided by 14 = .7142857

D   Remove the decimal point and put the percentage sign after the first two numbers

E   The answer is 71%

Unclear?

Grab your calculator and try one.
Pretend it is June 29th.
Jane started her 'year' of 'send positive notes to family members' on June 1st.

Every day since the 1st she has written a yes or no in her tracking journal.

She has 14 yes check marks.

What is her percentage?

Need Help?

A   29 days (Jane started her practice 29 days ago)

B   14 days (Jane tracked 'yes' that she sent out positive notes to family members)

C   14 divided by 29 = .48275

D   Remove the decimal point and put the percentage sign after the first two numbers

E   The answer is 48%

Reminder

Your 365 days begins when you decide. It is not a January 1st resolution. The day you launch and start tracking is considered your first day - the day you start counting **A**.

You don't have to wait 365 days to know how you're doing at any given time. It's vital to use the formula often (approximately weekly) to calculate your ongoing progress.

More Number Play

Let's say you love looking at the way numbers break down, and you also think doing something 201 days out of 365 seems ominous. Perhaps you even think—for a couple of your practices—that you know you won't want to do them on the weekends. Here's some number play for you. (In Jane's example, maybe she is not going to use her computer on weekends, therefore there are no notes going out on weekends.)

Start with 365 days. Tell yourself you do not ever have to do the practice on weekends. That eliminates 104 days immediately (52 weeks * 2 days).You can still hit 201 days. 365 minus 104 leaves 261 OPPORTUNITY days, so you still have 60 days that you don't have to practice. And you'll STILL be successful at 201. Pressure off.

For some people, on specific practices, this is a helpful solution. It gives a feeling of reduced stress. It highlights the message of 'choice'. Some of their practices they will want to do on the weekends, but for those things where there might be some fuss from the source—that being themselves—it's an option. It's doable.

PART III

Practicing

"To be re-inspired is to reconnect with, and to add to, your spectacular story."

Teresa Easler

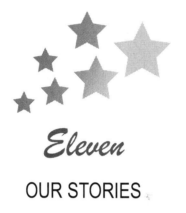

Eleven

OUR STORIES

Honesty

Judy M, holistic productivity guru of The Goddess Temple, has been referred to as the 'glue' on our team. She's facilitated the motivational calls in our pilot group, and is a social media miracle worker. Judy noted that there was a time she went on a business trip and 'fell off' practicing. This was not just on the trip, but for two weeks after she returned.

"I considered restarting instead of picking up where I left off. It was because of the numbers. But that wouldn't be honest. When I looked at my practices, I knew they were all real to me so I picked back up and counted, as in recorded, the days I'd not practiced. It was important that they be in my calculation."

Judy says that, having been part of the pilot group and their sharing, recommitment is normal.

"I believe people will go through a period where they stop and start (even if they're not going on a trip or vacation). It's part of the process. It might even be the Gremlin inside that emerges to stop us from doing something. That's why it's essential not to give up, and why it's really important not to start over from scratch. The final numbers will tell a story. That story needs to be truthful. In essence, that 'happily ever after' is 'freedom'."

Judy's advice on tracking is summarized as follows: Go to your heart. Don't cheat the system because the system is you. Be honest. Did you select the right choices for you? If so, then pick up and start recording again. This is a process of growth, of learning about yourself. Don't shut it out because the classroom of you is so important for your future and for the future of your community.

Judy has some wise words about the actual choices made.

"It's important to choose things that are fun, important to you, and 'well chosen' in that you've thought them out and truly asked yourself what it is you want. You may feel you 'should' lose weight, but you might *want* to be happier and that might look like losing weight, but is actually having a freer schedule. As a result, the weight might come off when you are happy because you are making better choices overall, or because your stress levels are reduced, or just maybe you are the right size for you and you just didn't realize it. Consider there are other things out there that you might not have thought out, or might have only dreamed about."

Judy's choices are unique—one could say they are customized for her, by her. She encourages creativity and thinking outside the box. One of her choices is something she called Morning Bliss. Based on *Miracle Morning* by Hal Elrod, her 'practice' comprises several things that are done in the morning—to start her day.

Another of Judy's practices was to spend time developing her intuition. She does this by going into her body and asking for the next step.

As she has said, the practices do not have to be conventional. The only 'should' is that the practices 'should' be tailored to what you want.

An example of a practice that will grow Judy and lead her to new heights within her personal and professional life is her practice of 'surrender'. Defined, it is to receive love and be a good receiver. She tracks this at the end of the day by looking back through the day and noting whether she was able to accept a compliment, recognize someone's caring toward her, and whether she gave love to herself.

She has a benevolent desire. "My wish is that 201 Day Achievement Principle is a vehicle to support people in realizing how simple it can be to be more fulfilled."

Two For One

Theresa M, our designer, experienced an interesting bonus with one of her practices. Perhaps you will notice some bonuses with yours.

Theresa had chosen meditation as one of her practices. Her intention was to do it in the morning. And that is exactly what she did. She enjoyed it immensely; it was an amazing start to her day. She tracked it. She chose the days. She felt great. Then she noticed she was waking earlier. She noted that one of the practices she had considered, but not chosen, was to get up earlier.

On observation she decided that the morning meditation practice was enjoyed and therefore buoyed her to rise early, yet the rising early—a consequence of the morning meditation—was also pleasurable and a win for her day.

She was thrilled that a practice had birthed a bonus. After a time, she wondered: was she now getting up early—because she enjoyed what that brought to her day—and then meditating, or was meditation still driving the getting up early?

Rising early and meditation became intertwined. Meditation supported getting up early. Getting up early supported meditation. Bonus!

Putting Back In

Founder, Kim White, had some thoughts in enhancing his regular practices: "So much of our practice mentality is to take things away and abstain. I decided to put something back in. In a mini practice for the 40 days of Lent, I decided, counter to taking something out, giving something up, I'd put something in. So I chose to do the Rosary every day."

Later on he spoke about tracking and practicing: "When we get good at stuff, then we think we don't have to be thinking of these things. Then we drop off. We realize, in hindsight, that we were good at those things because we kept note of doing those things—we kept a record of our practicing. This is really important to keep in mind because the power of tracking in the journal really supports our 'memory'."

*"What's different
about you is YOU."*

Teresa Easler

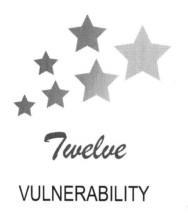

Twelve

VULNERABILITY

'Show and Tell' may well have introduced us to the world of sharing, but those were mostly simple times, and we were innocent voices. Somewhere along the line, many of us began to feel that sharing created a pressure to perform, brought about unwanted judgement, and even decided that when they did share successes they felt a bit boastful.

Some people are natural sharers and they are buoyed and motivated when they do. Their unbridled passion, nerves of steel, and resilience to negative talk is simply off the charts.

The act of sharing their plan motivates them to perform, to show that they can do it. Even when they stumble, their confidence allows them to pick right up where they left off—centre stage. Hey, there's nothing wrong with an audience if you're self-assured.

But guess what? When it comes to 201 Day Achievement Principle, there's nothing wrong with an audience either—especially when it's curated by you.

If you're naturally shy, or have been conditioned to keep your plans close to your chest, consider that, with careful planning, you can reap the rewards of putting yourself on the stage, and participate in the greater benefit of sharing, which is inspiring others.

Just as other people can inspire others to positive change, so can you inspire others.

Should You Share?

If you are considering sharing, decide if you will:

☆ **Share the generalities of 201 Day Achievement Principle.**

"Hey, there's this cool thing called 201 Day Achievement Principle."

☆ **Share a little more.**

"Hey, I'm doing some things in 201 Day Achievement Principle."

☆ **Share the practices you've chosen.**

"Guess what? I'm going to learn German."

☆ **Share the ongoing outcomes.**

"You know I set out to read that book series? Well this month I exceeded my target of reading. I'm currently at 65%."

☆ **Share to receive support.**

"I'm working to eat breakfast every day. Can you boil some eggs at night when you make supper?"

☆ **Share to give to other 'practice-ers' support in their pursuits.**

"I love that you're writing the book you always wanted to write. Want me to take the kids every Saturday morning?"

And consider the people you might share with (and why you're sharing):

☆ **A group of people you don't know who are doing 201 Day Achievement Principle.**

"Hey my name is 'MARY' and I'm happy to be a part of this Facebook group."

☆ **A close family member.**

"Sis, I want to tell you about something I'm working on. I'd like to keep it between us."

☆ **A friend.**

"Remember I said I always wanted to read War and Peace? Well I started."

☆ **A co-worker.**

"I'm headed to the gym right after work most days. I've made a goal for myself."

☆ **Someone who is already well versed in the practice you chose.**

"I so admire that you got your brown belt when you were in your forties. I wanted you to know I just joined a class."

You've Got This

When you share, access your wisdom, go over the reasons why you're sharing and then consider the person you're sharing with. Think about the guidelines around the share. Do you want them to tell others, or is it private? Don't assume. For example, it might be great that a co-worker knows you're headed to the gym after work. She'll understand why you're not hanging about or going for drinks. But, if you're taking a class in advanced-computer-genius-input with an eye to getting a promotion, then that might not be a great thing to share if you work in a competitive office.

Likewise, if you received negative messages from an older sibling, perhaps about the remedial reading you did in grade six, then you might not want to tell a chatty 'other sibling' about your goal of reading *War and Peace*.

Don't entertain any shares that could net you negative results. On the other hand, share your heart out when there is going to be celebration of you, accolades, support, and encouragement.

"*Frustration is the dynamic tension between what we commit to and what we experience. In times of frustration, take your attention to the 'what do I want to have happen?' Focus on the missing piece and the missing peace.*"

Teresa Easler

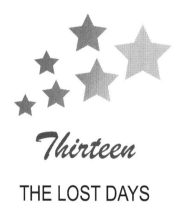

Thirteen

THE LOST DAYS

Hey, it's okay. On any journey there are stalls, delays, and setbacks. Sometimes there is 'stuff' on the tracks.

Lack of planning can be the cause of many a setback. Of course, the way to combat this is to plan. Everyone's heard the saying: Failing to plan is planning to fail.

Planning—being organized—is mainly a time issue. There are all kinds of sayings about time: *I don't have enough. Where did it go? Wow, look at the time! I've run out of time. I'll do it later. Sorry I'm late. I need a time machine.*

Clock Time And Recalibration

Time is delivered, second by second, sunrise by sunrise, in the same increments for every living soul. The way we allocate our time—the choices we make to spend our time—is what sets us apart.

Clock time that marks days, nights, weeks, months, years, and lifetimes, does not have to be an enemy. For as long as rudimentary calendars have been in existence, we've all adhered to timetables. Each one of us can either fight against it or learn to thrive within it by living in the now.

That does not mean that you will never be able to relax or enjoyably lose track of time.

It is inevitable that pockets of real-time are swallowed up each day by appointments, classes, work-hours, and sleep. Though folks tend to believe these are non-negotiable, and certainly attending a class from two o'clock until three-thirty *is* set in stone, there are swaths of time between scheduled hours that are unscheduled. These hours are available but people choose to let them slide. How many times have you been on social media, descended into the rabbit hole, and come out the other side forty five minutes later? It's common to think, "Wow, I could have walked a mile and made supper by now."

This is not to say that time on social media is not fun, desired, supportive, connection-centred, enjoyable, even educational, but the way you pass your time is a choice. Many a time people have complained that they didn't have enough time to write that essay, start that book, knit that sweater, go for a walk, or wash their hair, all the while ignoring the time 'wasted' by gossiping about Jane's affair, debating about the latest political issues, or posting pictures of puppies.

We create a clock around our lives.
We can recalibrate that clock at any time.

There is no need to be superman and fly around the world to reverse time. Sure, it would be great to get back some of those past moments—to have a few re-do's. But since life is not a super-hero fantasy, it's important to be present and make things happen in the now. In order to use the 24 hours a day to your advantage you simply need to analyze, choose, and recalibrate. In other words, reallocate. The goal is to be master of the clock, not let the clock be the master. What that really means is to take an honest look at what you do throughout the day.

What you might find upon analysis—reviewing one day/being mindful of how one day is spent—is that there is time wasted or squandered, and time not used efficiently. Note: time management is not meant to turn you into a robot.

Here are some things that steal your days:

☆ Keeping Facebook open in the background creates mini-breaks that add up to maxi-minutes, then become hours.

☆ Checking email randomly. It's better to take 2, 3, or 4 scheduled times to check and prioritize replies.

☆ Avoiding the 'task' that is least liked. You'd be surprised how liberating it is to get rid of that 'task' first thing. You'd be shocked at how avoidance is basically a foot-tapping exercise that generates, well, more foot tapping.

☆ Multitasking. This is really convincing yourself you can do more than one thing at one time. 'Multitasking' simply creates chaos and the 'tasks' take much longer or go unfinished. Not to mention that the level of error goes up when a single focus becomes corrupted with an effort to multi-focus.

Recalibrating your personal schedule does not mean overscheduling or crossing out downtime. On the contrary, it is freeing. Owning your own time means coming face to face with your lifestyle. It means throwing away the way you've thought your schedule MUST be, and taking a blank page and comparing what you 'think you do' and what you 'actually do' and then evaluating what you 'want to do and also need to do'. Many people find that when they are serious about recalibrating, they have been operating within an inefficient system.

For example, a freelance writer believed she needed to work every day and night in order to get all her jobs and projects finished on time. When she kept track of her days, she realized that flexibility had allowed her to get up at nine, sometimes ten, be at her desk at noon, and then feel like a slave when she was still at her desk at night. When she recalibrated, she discovered she was able to complete all her work in a focused thirty-five hours a week. What had been a destructive pattern—she'd allowed flexibility to squander large blocks of time—soon righted itself to a sane schedule.

There was more than enough time. She simply had to take a look at what she was doing, and how what she was doing had become a part of her belief system.

Again, the key is to look honestly at how you spend your time—to carve out specific times for what you want to do, including down time, and to be the master of the clock. That begins with understanding that we all have the same amount of time, that we probably do things that are totally unnecessary, that there are probably more efficient ways to do things, and that our attitude around 'time' has been corrupted by the 'busy-must-be-everything-to-everyone' mindset.

Many believe that wearing 'busy' as a badge of honour elevates them among their peers. It's an easy trap to fall into. 'People will think more of me if I work sixty hours a week. People will think less of me if I appear to have a lot of free time.'

Overscheduled adults, and overscheduled children, are rarely happy people.

Down time and balance is healthy, and downright sexy. Recalibration allows people to observe their schedules and take control of their lives.

Teresa E's Recalibration - Salon Solution

"Recently, at the salon, I anticipated a rather long appointment. I was lamenting that I had not been meditating as often as I wanted to. It struck me that the timing was perfect. I could tune out and create a meditation slot right in the chair. It was simple. And it wasn't multitasking since I had nothing to do with the styling. So, I closed my eyes. And off I went. Later on, when I opened my eyes, the stylist asked me: 'Teresa, were you meditating?' "

Theresa M's Recalibration - Refining

Theresa M is a busy mom who was creative when she redefined her exercise goals as PLAY MORE. She also discovered the bonus of rising early when she practiced meditation.

One of her other 'wants' which she decided to track as a practice was to work on her business more than she was. She was actively working 'in' her business, but felt she needed to do more work 'on' the business. When she'd narrowed this, she decided an hour would be a 'session' that would warrant a 'yes I've practiced'. As a result of tweaking the time, she felt empowered by the amount of yeses she recorded in her journal.

"Well, it turned out I did work on my business, but one hour was too long. My life revolves around children's naps and kindergarten. I set a shorter time, and felt much more in control of my schedule."

The Saboteur Within AKA Let's Stop Now Before You Waste Your Time

You know her as the Gremlin, the Inner-saboteur; perhaps you've called her the Green Monster. She might even be known as Ms. McFaultfinder. Her sole mission in your life is to destroy your dreams. Well, that sounds a little severe but, sadly, for some, it is true.

Many people have theorized and written about the Inner-saboteur.

One theory is that, basically, evolution has developed within us a protector (who would have thought this Gremlin was on our side?). This protector is a leftover in our programming from the days when it was important to have an inner-sense of 'don't do it'. Life was high-risk in a predatory world. But we don't live in the wild any longer, with hungry prey in the shadows.

Another explanation theorizes that we received messages in the past—childhood—and because of those messages there is now an impairment in our belief system (belief in ourselves), and that our Inner-saboteur comes to save us from successes we fear we can't sustain.

In Debi Silber's TEDx talk on why we sabotage ourselves, change—and the fear of what we are going to do or be—along with peers not liking our changing, explains 'giving up and abandoning new directions'. Her passionate speech outlines the way people get into realization, experience the joy of the change, and then quickly retreat.

These are extremely simplified takes. Further study would lead one to the subject of the ego about which there are many brilliant studies and books.

**The Gremlin is ever-present and shows
up at crucial times, uninvited.**

Though she's no longer needed—people are grown-ups and mostly confident in their pursuits—she still shows. But folks don't need her doubting voice. And to say the Inner-sab is a doubting voice is putting it mildly.

The point for this section is to give you a few tools for dealing with that monster who rises and puts you down, incites doubt, laughs at you for attempting something.

The good news is the more you 'deal' with her from a logical standpoint, the less she shows up.

The best way to handle your Inner-sab may sound counter-intuitive, but it is to shine the spotlight on her. It is to be aware. As soon as you are aware of her presence, you are in a position of power.

Awareness is the beginning of the answer.

When you hear the voice of doubt, stop for a moment. Give it a few seconds in the spotlight and truly listen. Listen to the words. How ridiculous do they sound? Compare them with your intent and your strength. Imagine them spoken from your own mouth to one of your mentors, or to a friend. Would they make sense? Imagine a trusted friend or family member saying them to you. Beyond ridiculous, huh?

Let's take a couple of 'examples' of what might be heard from an Inner-sab. Think about how cruel, hurtful, damaging, and outrageous they sound.

Kathleen is creating the outline to a book she plans to write about people being able to maintain their own vehicle.

The voice comes just as she types the first point. "Who the hell do you think you are? You're no writer."

On examination, would you say that to anyone? Would you ever have said that to the author of your favourite book? What about to a small child who has set about writing what he did on his summer vacation? Of course not.

The awareness Kathleen can apply when she hears that statement is powerful. She needs first to acknowledge the Inner-sab's statement, and that it is a cruel thing. Then she needs to assure herself this is not true.

It's important Kathleen not defend or argue. It's best for Kathleen to distance herself from the voice. Sure, there could be a lot of analysis on why Kathleen's Inner-sab said this. It could even go back to when she wrote about her own summer vacation and the grade four bully who taunted her. This is not a time for Kathleen to analyze. It is a time for Kathleen to act.

The best thing Kathleen can do is step back, give the Inner-sab the floor, and take a look at it. What colour is this character? What shape? What does the Inner-sab look like?

Then, Kathleen can make a mental list of her own true self—the true Kathleen. Kathleen is the head mechanic at a car dealership. Her father was a mechanic too. Kathleen is a benevolent person. Kathleen loves to write. Kathleen has an editor friend who is going to look over her first draft.

When Kathleen's Inner-sab visits her, it is the perfect time for Kathleen to remind herself of all the above, and her intention: that she knows people who struggle with money, and that she wants to help them avoid costly mechanical bills.

She can recall how the owner of the dealership told her she was a champion, and congratulated her for her plan to donate a bunch of her books to a community organization that helps people purchase cars.

By this time, if the Inner-sab hasn't already left, Kathleen can confidently dismiss the monster.

Note: It will take practice. The Inner-sab doesn't leave lightly. The Inner-sab takes on the qualities of a nosey neighbour, always dropping in with a pie baked with salt instead of sugar. The Inner-sab lurks behind a flimsy curtain.

Kathleen's—and therefore your—awareness and treatment is tantamount to installing privacy blinds.

The Inner-sab loses power when you exercise awareness. That is, stop, listen, apply the statement to those you love, and affirm your position. The Inner-sab shrinks from benevolence and humanitarian endeavours.

Gremlins often show up in lifestyle-change initiatives. What that means is they barge in when we're dieting.

On ordering an ice cream cone, this was the horrible statement made by the Inner-sab: "Darlene, you fat cow, you'll never lose weight."

Stop. Listen. That is so mean. And it's unfounded. How does that Inner-sab know Darlene will never lose weight?

Darlene needs to ask herself: "Would I say that to my best friend?" She needs to speak the statement in her mind, with her friend's name: "Susan my friend, you fat cow, you will never lose weight." She can try it out this way too: "Mom, you fat cow, you will never lose weight." This will affirm for Darlene how horrid the statement is. It will let her know that this statement isn't worthy of any acceptance. It is cruel and it is ridiculous.

If this happens to you—or when it does—and when you've stopped and listened, then reaffirm YOUR intentions. "I've been tracking my 201 out of 365 days on abstinence from dairy, and on less than 25 grams of carbs a day. I am in the 60% range for each. This is a choice. I am a human being, and a human deserving of balance. I am already losing weight and, as a bonus, I am understanding lifestyle balance." When you feel confident, return to the Inner-sab and ask her to leave (she may have already darted away, sensing defeat).

Overzealousness

It's a mouthful. And it's an unusual one. But it is true, overzealousness can cause setbacks.

This happens when the freedom of the choice of when to practice (keeping in mind 201 days out of 365 is a target) becomes frantic fanaticism (a leaning to want to have a one-hundred percent streak).

201 Day Achievement Principle was created to bring success to those who practice consistently and realistically.

Some high-achievers, or those folks high on the idea of change, experience a bit of obsession. Overdoing things usually leads to burnout.

Can you see how this might happen?

Here's what might appear to be an extreme creation to example overzealousness. 'Bob' is going to learn martial arts. It's something he wanted to do as a boy. He signs up for a class. He worries he will not be in shape for the class, so he signs up for additional fitness to support his initial plan. Then, in week one, he discovers he's not that flexible—the instructor tells him it'll come in time, but Bob is set on that belt program, and feels 'authentic' wearing the karate-whites (he wants his skill to match his karategi—that's the outfit aka a gi) that he joins yoga to get flexible. His 201 days of 365 with the practice of getting involved in martial arts has now stretched to fill five out of seven nights of classes. He pushes himself for four weeks. Then he begins to forget what he originally started this for. He even sprains his ankle in a high-impact aerobics drop-in he thought would help him with stamina. Six weeks after he had chosen his practice and entered YES in his tracking journal he is defeated.

It's not just in exercise. A person could just as well have chosen to learn to knit and intend to have a sweater completed by the end of 365 days. You got it: in the overzealous scenario, the freedom of taking up knitting, and the imagining knitting while watching a movie, becomes fanatical. From 'wow, I can cast on the stitches' to, 'look, I did four rows without dropping a stitch', the obsession grows. Pretty soon, the knitter is dreaming about the clicking of knitting needles—it's all she sees. The practice is no longer fun. The sweater has become a must-do-at-all-costs.

Avoid the 'overzealous' setback by setting reasonable targets. After all, 201 days out of 365 days is the perfect example of reasonable.

Illness

Sickness can be a downfall. There's nothing like a nasty flu to create a backslide, a series of days not participated/days not marked yes. You are human. It's okay. Begin with some forgiveness and cut yourself some slack.

Remember how we said planning is a great thing? Well, when you are well, without becoming fanatical, do some extra days to raise your percentages. Basically, what we promote is to bank days. Put in a little extra effort, when you are healthy, to anticipate and provide coverage for times when you are under the weather.

Work/Travel

Travel for work can also disrupt participation in practice. A heavy travel schedule calls for innovation.

Teresa E'S Story

The Curse of the Mat, The Power of having Shared, and a Happily Ever After Solution

"Travel is a huge component of my work. Yoga is one of my practices. I love it. It's a part of my life. But the bulk of the mat—even though it's quite thin—created issues for me at the airport. I ended up not traveling with it. When I arrived at my destination, I found hotel towels to be too slippery and, whether the floor was carpeted, tiled, or hardwood, I found it difficult to practice. Thank goodness I'd shared my practice and my dilemma with a friend (there is power in sharing). She presented the solution by finding the most unusual things I had ever seen: yoga socks and yoga gloves. I didn't know they existed. They pack easily, and prevent me from slipping on any surface. Work travel is no longer a setback for my practice of yoga."

Vacation

As much as you might think you can take your 'goal' of reading Ulysses on vacay, you might prefer 'Hawaiian Affair' for a summer read on the beach. Allow for what you want to do, and do not want to do, on vacation.

If Yoga is your practice, and you're going on a yoga retreat, then that's a bonus—you're sure to be tracking it. But if you're going to Vegas with a pile of friends for an all-out party-fest, then it's doubtful you'll be doing yoga.

Consider putting in some extra time toward your practices a few weeks before you go away.

If you know your vacation will not support your practice, then the month before you leave for a family reunion, step up the online French lessons; that way your percentage will be on target when you get back.

Knowing how to prevent, avoid, or get through delays and set-backs generates a sense of power. Take a look at your schedule. Decide when you know you will not be in any position to participate and track your practice.

We know you can't decide when you might be ill, but you likely do know that you have a business conference the week of June 23rd, or you will be caring for a relative the weekend of the 10th. Advance plan. Anticipate. There's success in that.

Success generates enthusiasm. Take that enthusiasm and use it for good.

Monkeying Around

When we created the pilot group we Survey Monkeyed them when they were a little bit into their journey. We wanted to know what obstacles they encountered so that we could offer support to them, and ensure 201 Day Achievement Practice would be fully developed when it went live.

Though most reported they were on target, enjoying the freedom, and loving this new way of looking at their progress and growth, a small percentage did report a setback or two.

We categorized these or defined these as limiting beliefs. And we brainstormed and consulted participants to find solutions to these limiting beliefs.

Self-Limiting Belief One - External

It was noted that the external limiting belief was related to the use of the tracking journal. Some found it challenging to track things. It was a limiting belief because participants were not used to using paper journals, schedulers, or trackers.

If you're not used to using journals, know that it takes time to get used to something new. To make it easier, do everything you can to make it convenient. This includes:

☆ Have the journal and a pen together. Pens are like socks and Tupperware lids: often missing in action.

☆ Have the pen and the journal in a handy place where you will see it every day. Bedside table, in your bag with your phone, on the music stand, in the bathroom. Whatever works for you.

☆ Link the practice of recording with something else that you do rote, like brushing teeth, prayer, before-bed glass of water, nighttime gratitude list.

☆ Consider that the element of having support for your
practices will drive you to record your participation. Talking
yourself through the 'why' you are using the journal is all that
is needed to overcome the belief that you can't or won't use
it

It is because of tracking that you will achieve results.

Hikers would bring a water bottle on a hike. Yoga-folks would
bring a yoga mat to yoga class. Participants in 201 Day Achievement
Principle bring their tracking journal with them, or have it handy.

Hikers drink from the water bottle (and fill it and wash it). It's
vital to their enjoyment of the hike. Yoga-folks lie on the yoga mat
and enjoy the padding. The water bottle and the yoga mat support
the success of the hike or the yoga session. It's the same for the
tracking journal. It's a tool that supports the success.

*Remember how Natalie put her tracking journal on her bedside
table and brought tracking into her nighttime ritual?

Restating The Belief:
"Making tracking simple drives my journey to success."

Self-Limiting Belief Two - Internal

We asked about internal struggles with following through. Most
said that there was no internal struggle. However, there were some
people who said, "Nothing ever sticks. I've tried so many things
before. I will probably forget to track."

"I'm not good enough." "I tried this kind of thing before." "It's
hard for me to stick with something."

If you are one of these people, then it's time to think back to
your story. To think about what and why you chose 'in the past'
and how 'this time' is different. And it is different. There has never

been a program like the 201 Day Achievement Principle; a program where you are not asked to do something for one hundred percent of the time.

It is important to consider how 'this time' you are more prepared to succeed, and that 201 days out of 365 is totally doable, and that anything less than that, as long as you are tracking, is also a win.

☆ **Reminding yourself to be gentle with yourself is vital.**

☆ **Remembering that you are in a program that is gentle with you is essential.**

☆ **201 Daily Achievement Principle promotes slow and steady; it understands human nature, and gets how your past can influence your future.**

Do the best you can to release the 'before' and focus on the now. Imagine being accountable to yourself for the first time in your life. And imagine that accountability supporting you to be kind to yourself. Review the 'freedom' associated with choosing to participate in the practice you selected.

Perhaps this is the first time you've ever been prepared for success. Celebrate that.

It's totally okay to tell yourself you are worthy of whatever participation you choose.

Remember what Camille said about her process? She chose her practices by framing them with, 'I wanted to hold my own hand.'

Restating The Belief:
"It starts with being my own best friend, and that involves believing in myself."

Self-Limiting Belief Three – Follow Through

The final limiting belief we covered with the pilot group was the external struggle of follow through.

Many felt that an accountability partner would help—and we answered that by providing a Facebook group. Many a friend-match can be made, one that is even closer than in the general group. There are people doing what you are doing. There are people doing things you may not have ever thought of. Your practice may be interesting to other people. What everyone has in common on the Facebook group is that they are maximizing the outcome of success. Sharing and support is proven to boost participation.

Time was another factor, and we've covered this in clock time. Time is a factor in most everything you do. That said, it does not have to be a negative factor. Being the master of time has the reward of feeling accomplished and in control of life. For those who felt that writing in the tracking journal took too much time, we reminded that a simple yes or no would work—no one is expected to write a novel—the app would surely assist in the time issue. That said, there is value in pen to paper, and some say that the more consistently they record—and add their feelings—the more successful they feel and the more accomplished they become.

*Remember we have talked about our Facebook page? Support awaits you. As for time: let flexibility be your friend—remember, you set the time limit for your participation in your practice.

Restating The Belief:
"Support is as close as a click on my phone."
"Everyone has the same 24 hours in a day."

TAKEAWAYS

★ Never underestimate the power of planning.

★ Awareness stops an Inner-sab in its tracks.

★ Banking days provides an awesome advantage.

LISTENING IN ON THE THOUGHTS OF OTHERS
INTERJECTION/EXCERPT:
A PARTICIPANT SHARES

"I know I am quite an all or nothing person. I like the way the book stated that 201 Day Achievement Principle is a whole other place, different than all or nothing but, on reading the part about being overzealous, I can see me all over that. It's been my downfall in the past. So I decided to go over what I'd learned so far in the book. And I thought about the niching. I thought it might be really good for me to niche my practice or practices because if I ended up with ten niches from one practice that would show me I'd bitten off more than I could chew. Next, I thought that niching might make me feel that there was enough on my plate—I like seeing lists and categories and breakdowns. If I saw more words I might ease up on adding more activities related to the practice. Then I realized that this is different than any other 'program' I've tried. I told myself that if I was going to introduce myself to new concepts, I might as well add 'reasonable expectations' to that list. For the first time in my life I found myself giving 'me' advice that I often give others. "Be Gentle With Yourself." I know my own quirks, and I can see me just bar-relling into a practice and expanding it to the point of my burning out. BUT!!!! It's a big but. For the first time ever I'm anticipating it. And so by foreseeing it, I can stop it. Awareness is power."

FAQ's

I keep coming back to that difference. Aren't they really the same thing? Practice and Habit. Isn't it like some say tom-AY-to and some say tom-ah-to?

It may be that you're getting tripped up on 'if a practice is done enough that it becomes a habit'. And that can absolutely happen, but it would take a lot longer than 201 out of 365 days. Let's go over it again. It's a great question. **Habits** are associated with being automatic, and they are not always something that is 'enjoyed' or even 'good for us'. (Think the good: brushing teeth. Think the not so good: picking at mosquito bites.) **A practice** is freely chosen, and it is something that is always 'wanted'. When you think practice, think passion. When you think habit, think 'rote'.

I'm an introvert. More than an introvert. My practices are super-private. Three out of my four are what I deem 'not share-able'. Two of them have to do with moving away from something extremely negative. How can I benefit from the rewards—physical and mental—that are described here, and yet remain anonymous?

The power is all yours. You have an absolute right to keep your practices private. That said, there is great benefit from being cheered on. Would you be willing to join the Facebook page—**201 Day Achievement Principle**—and share your progress without naming the practice? People will respect your entries, and still encourage you and cheer you on, regardless of you not identifying the actual practice. That said, can you check in with yourself to ensure you are not feeling that you will be ridiculed because of your choices (if they were exposed) or that you are not feeling shame, and have chosen a mindset around your practices which generate more shame for you? Privacy is one thing. Shrouding one's opportunity for growth in mystery—and in particular mystery laced in shame—is another. If you are clear after that, then consider the number labels. And, please be gentle with yourself. You know you. If you can find a way to step a little bit out of your comfort zone, then fantastic. That might look like a circle on your calendar and a 'name' for your start date; it might mean a cup of tea and a quiet corner; perhaps you could make yourself a play-list to represent the success you anticipate—then listen to your playlist (privately) as a celebration and recognition of your milestones.

YOUR SPACE FOR YOUR NOTES

Can you release any concerns that you will not measure up? Can you summarize those concerns in a word and write a positive word to counter each concern?

Can we just say how much we want you to succeed. Why do you want to succeed?

"Positive thoughts are not enough. You need passion, commitment, and action."

Kim White

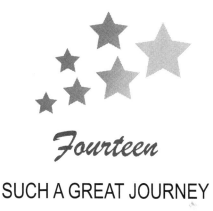

Fourteen

SUCH A GREAT JOURNEY

At the beginning of this book we said that train tracks lead to chosen destinations—exotic and exciting places awaiting your arrival. Well, you're aboard and on your way to success via the 201 Day Achievement Principle.

By choosing to read this book, you've chosen *not* to take the express route. Instead, you've opened yourself to view the full landscape of learning about you and how you look at choice, tracking, and success. You're holding a Golden Ticket, and you'll use it throughout the year to access all kinds of amazing places that will provide dozens of interesting feelings.

Three hundred and sixty-five days from the start of your 'year' you will arrive in a new place as a changed you.

In wrapping up all we've touched on in this book, we want to give you a few last tips to make the next part of your journey the best it can be.

☆ **We want for you to be the missing piece in your own life.**
Breathe and break – you will be so much more successful for having down-time so that you are present for yourself.

☆ **Be gentle with yourself.**
Words matter. For example: 'spending time in nature' is a more meaningful and specific statement than 'get exercise'.

☆ **"Be impeccable with your word."** Don Miguel Ruiz (*The Four Agreements*):
And when you are impeccable with your word, make sure that includes your self-talk.

☆ **Be respectful to yourself.**
We still consider you a contributor. We ask you now: What does being respectful to yourself mean? What 'words' will you need to drop? What words will you need to use?

As a participant and contributor to this book and to 201 Day Achievement Principle you become a practitioner in your own life—can you call yourself that? How about an Architect of Life or an Interior Designer? Remember, words matter, and role-taking can drive and motivate. What will you call yourself?

Imagine you have a crystal ball in front of you. Project where you believe one, two, or all of your chosen practices will take you?

Think about your belief in yourself. Keep 'you' in your thoughts.

☆ **You will experience change, you will evoke it in others.**
As you change, there may be some resistance from others; they're used to the old you. Be patient with them, but do not let 'their' discomfort alter your path.

What do you need from yourself to be fully supported? It can be something as simple as:

☆ An alarm clock.

☆ The kettle filled with water before you go to bed.

☆ A packed lunch the night before.

☆ A reminder from a friend or family member that you are loved.

☆ Less contact with someone.

☆ More contact with someone else.

☆ Extra pens.

☆ A walking buddy.

☆ An accountability partner.

☆ A journal.

☆ An app to record your monologues.

☆ A knapsack...

... you get the idea.

Regardless of whether these 'helping things' are for your heart and soul, your brain, or your physical body, honouring them will move you toward success.

Fill that kettle and put your best teacup beside it. Make sure to have the ingredients for good packed lunches, and allocate the time to prepare it when you do your dinner. Ask your bestie to call you each week to tell you some good news, or to remind you of something valuable about you.

Have you everything in place to be fully supported on this journey? What are a few simple things you can adjust to create more room for success?

☆ Reminder: You own your own time.

We said at the beginning of this book:

We mostly approach things alone and throw ourselves into them rather than have structure. 201 Day Achievement Principle is different than any other program you've encountered. No one is demanding one hundred percent participation. The fact that no one is demanding stringent perfection means you are likely to arrive at your year end as a changed person. You are choosing your goals and the amount of time you will practice in each session, as well as when you will practice. You hold all the power.

Are you clear on that? Is there leftover 'competitive-streak energy' from other programs? If you have any concerns, engage with other participants, send us an email, reframe them to live outside that concern or those concerns, get creative—use those concerns as a catalyst for change—and thrive.

Sound Advice

If you crater, stop, or experience any setback, step outside yourself and look at the situation from a distance. The world didn't end. More importantly, the program—your program—didn't end. Your stall might not be for the 'worst' but for the 'change' and change always contains at least one message. Take the time to have a conversation with yourself, interview yourself aloud in a monologue, and record it on your phone if you like. There will be lessons and messages in that depth of conversation. What you thought was a setback is just change. It can be modified to create even more success.

Invest in yourself. Take your Golden Ticket and create a golden life. Yes, it's that doable. It may seem like two or four practices that you consider 'small' cannot possibly be life-changing. They are important to you for well-thought-out reasons. They may well lead you to other things you truly want.

Cross country trips are achieved by facing in the right direction and moving one kilometre at a time. Big dreams are achieved by accomplishing smaller tasks.

This year you may come out at 41% on sewing. Next year you may be 87%. The following year you might be creating kimonos for a local theatre company in NYC. This is the power of choosing practices and tracking consistently.

It's like getting on a train and journeying to the place you know you belong.

Yes, this seemingly simple platform is perhaps the most powerful action and impactful journey you will ever take.

Congratulations on all the learning about yourself you have done so far, and our heartfelt support for all the days of this year, and all years.

Link everything you do with love.

Is there anything that doesn't appeal to you at this point? Anything that is confusing? Do you need to go back over the math? Do an example here?

A *How many days since you started?*

B *How many days have you practiced?*

C *Take your number of days practiced (B) and divide by (A) the number of days since you started.*

D *On your calculator this will show you a decimal point and a 'number'.*

E *Remove the decimal before the number and place a percentage sign after the first two numbers.*

Example

A *14 days (I started 14 days ago)*

B *10 days (I have practiced – tracked YES in the journal)*

C *10 divided by 14 = .7142857*

D *Remove the decimal point and put the percentage sign after the first two numbers*

E *The answer is 71%*

ADDENDUM:
NODS, SHOUT-OUTS, AND WAVES

A little bit of back of book to seal our commitment, grow our relationship with you, and honour the process.

☆ Time Travel

☆ Further Ideas

☆ More Of Us

☆ Full Hearts

☆ Some of Our Sources

TIME TRAVEL

Can you imagine what it's going to feel like next year? You're going to read this:

**CONGRATULATIONS, HAPPY ANNIVERSARY.
WE ARE THRILLED THAT YOU COMPLETED A YEAR.**

Yes, you're going to hear from us. Please register with us so that we can keep in touch—send us an email to tell us the start date of your 'year' and be sure to share what your practices are—we want to keep 'track' of you. We're all on this journey together. Email us at: **201dayachievementprinciple@connecttothecore.com**

When your year is over, or any time during your year, take the time to think about how the program changed your way of thinking, then share it with us. Ask yourself what parts of the program were helpful. Go over if there's anything you did that made it even more doable, anything to improve the program. Share that with us so that we can grow too.

Celebrate your numbers, no matter what they are. Every number is worthy of celebration. Had you not started this one year ago you may never have achieved any progress.

Checklist for your year end:

☆ Have I planned a celebration/anniversary?

☆ Have I shared that this is a year end?
Will I do this again?

☆ If I am doing this again, will I keep the same practices?

☆ Which will I not keep?

☆ Will I add new ones?

☆ Have I thought about new ones?

☆ What will my new practices be?

☆ Will there be more or less?

☆ Have I planned a new launch?

☆ What was the most challenging thing about 201 Day Achievement Principle?

☆ How have I grown in each practice over this year?

☆ What have I noticed about myself as a result of the entire process?

FURTHER IDEAS FOR 201 DAY ACHIEVEMENT PRINCIPLE

This book and journal set would be a fantastic addition to anyone's personal growth toolbox. Be the catalyst for others by gifting or suggesting this book to:

☆ School staff associations

☆ Classrooms or groups of students: band, French class, drama club

☆ Business/Management: for the personal development of their employees

☆ Group homes: staff, residents, or both

☆ Organizations: Guides / Scouts

☆ Large family groups / Extended family groups / Family reunions

☆ Professional organizations

☆ Moms' groups

☆ Hobbyist organizations

LET US KNOW WHAT GROUPS YOU'VE SHARED WITH SO WE CAN CHEER THEM ON

MORE OF US

Take Us From The Page To The Stage

We are each available, in person or through the magic of media, to present to your organization or as keynotes or contributors at events. Specifically, in 2019, Kim—from Australia—marks his twenty-fifth anniversary of spiritual coaching and guidance, an international career spanning North and Central America, Europe, Asia, and the Southern Hemisphere: Australia and New Zealand. (**https://kimwhitecoaching.com**). And Teresa—Toronto, Canada—regularly works her magic throughout North America, in cross-country assignments for her firm, Connect To The Core. Solution oriented, she has been promoting and teaching excellence in communication for over thirty years (**https://connecttothecore.com**).

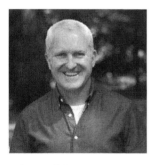

Kim White

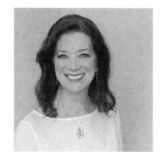

Teresa Easler

FULL HEARTS

Our heartfelt gratitude to everyone who contributed to making this book a life-changer for all.

- ☆ NATALIE - Your ability to wrangle entrepreneurs and keep a project and all its pieces moving forward is amazing. Thank you for your contribution in making this happen.

- ☆ JUDY – You are the glue in stellar project management. Beautiful becomes you. Your knowledge of the online world is marvelous.

- ☆ SHANNON – Queen of laughter and wit, your enthusiasm is contagious. You consistently bring up good points and bring us back to Earth.

- ☆ THERESA M – Creativity dances around you. You are the wow factor.

- ☆ CAMILLE— You are the contribution rock star—your ideas shine.

- ☆ MARIE – Your ability to capture, process and organize all of our crazy ideas and put them in one book is extraordinary.

SOME OF OUR SOURCES

https://www.health.harvard.edu/blog/your-well-being-more-than-just-a-state-of-mind-201303065957

https://www.precisionnutrition.com/body-transformation-research

https://hbr.org/ (Multiple articles: Harvard business review)

https://www.sciencedaily.com/releases/2015/10/151029101349.htm

https://www.intelligentchange.com/blogs/news (Multiple articles)

https://mayoclinichealthsystem.org/hometown-health/speaking-of-health/setting-smart-goals

https://www.nhs.uk/conditions/stress-anxiety-depression/raising-low-self-esteem/

https://www.psychologytoday.com/us/blog/evolution-the-self/201101/self-sabotage-and-your-outer-child-pt-4-5

https://www.encyclopedia.com/psychology/dictionaries-thesauruses-pictures-and-press-releases/antilibidinal-egointernal-saboteur

http://www.selfication.com/motivation/the-power-of-small-wins/

https://www.youtube.com/watch?v=XX3oi6nC7ro

Printed in Great Britain
by Amazon